THE ULTIMATE RECIPE FOR AN ENERGETIC LIFE

Simple Steps to Eating Well
And Feeling Your Best

KATHY Parry
Your Real Food Coach

The Ultimate Recipe for an Energetic Life

Simple Steps to Eating Well and Feeling Your Best

A Kathy Parry Book

Book Cover by Tracey Miller | www.TraceOfStyle.com
Publishing by Weston Lyon | www.WestonLyon.com
Edited by Lauren Cullumber

ISBN:1494737981
EAN-13: 978-1494737986

Disclaimer:

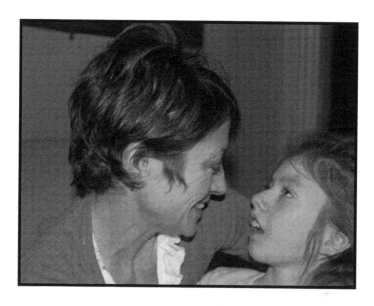

To Merritt Joy
You have very little energy, yet you radiate love
You have no words, yet you've told a story

All my love

The Ultimate Recipe for an Energetic Life

Table of Contents

Read This First!

Do you need caffeine and chocolate to make it through your day? Are you dragging by mid-afternoon? Unfocused? Unproductive? You're not alone. Millions of people feel tired and sluggish – even worn down – on a daily basis. The Ultimate Recipe for an Energetic Life gives you the information you need and desire to finally feel vital and productive!

Inside you will learn:

- The six simple steps you must take to live an energetic and engaged life!

- How to uncover the foods you're eating right now that are wreaking havoc on your body and keeping you tired all day long!

- Easy, delicious, and healthful recipes that will save you time and boost your energy levels so you can not only "keep up" – you can speed up!

- Success habits you can change TONIGHT to feel rested and ready-to-go tomorrow morning!

Each chapter teaches you important information about how you are sabotaging your energy levels, while giving you tips and tactics to combat these habits. You'll receive action steps that will give you a starting point for change. AND...each chapter includes delicious, healthful recipes designed for busy people.

I wrote this book because I am constantly asked how I stay energetic. As a business owner and mother of four, I'm passionate about helping others discover their ultimate energy and live a full life – and now I'm ready to share my secrets with you!

Are you ready to live an active and engaged life? A life full of passion, zest, and unlimited energy? With just a few changes, some fun stories and delicious recipes you'll be on your way. Let's get started!

Chapter 1
Wake Up

"To be awake is to be alive."
Henry David Thoreau

Get Your Head Off the Desk... And I'm Not Talking to Your Student!

When I was in junior high my history teacher fell asleep at his desk. While our heads hovered over a quiz on the Civil War, his head slowly slumped. And, before the bell rang, his face was plastered to his lesson plan. Snickering as we turned in our papers, we pointed and laughed at the drool slipping out of the corner of his mouth. Mr. Decker's lack of energy left him with the unfortunate nickname that would take him years to shake: Mr. Dribbles.

You Don't Want to Be Mr. Dribbles

I get it. My teacher was tired. What teacher isn't? They rise early, way too early, and they must stay energetic and focused all day. And the kids. Your own kids, the multitude of kids you're responsible for, and the adults who often act like kids, all draining you of energy. How is a teacher to keep his cheek from hitting the desk? How is a mom who runs around with toddlers going to be able to stay awake at work? Is a jet-lagged, nutrient-deprived salesperson going to be truly engaged in life? And how is a college student who is studying and partying ever going to make it through finals? All of them need to maintain energy! And we do this by treating our cells with respect.

9

Can You Get the Science Teacher Down Here?

Okay, forget just for a minute that science wasn't your favorite subject; it's time for a basic lesson in cells. Every one of your 75 trillion cells (your number may be closer to 50 trillion, especially if you killed off a few in college) produces energy in a cycle known at the Krebs cycle. Your cells daily convert food to energy. The mitochondria in your cells are the organisms that convert the food into ATP, the usable form of energy. If your cells are functioning at peak performance levels, you produce energy efficiently. But there are many reasons why we don't produce energy efficiently, and this book will examine some of these reasons. So why do I, as a mother of four, know and care about mitochondria and energy? Well, my fourth child got me schooled.

I Got Schooled

Happily pregnant with my fourth child, I was preparing organic, whole foods for my seven year old, five year old and two year old at home. A bit apprehensive as to how adding one more child to this highly energetic crew would work, I forged ahead waiting for our last child to arrive. Merritt Joy was born August 26, 2001. When Merritt was about nine weeks old, right around Thanksgiving, she began to do something that looked like an exaggerated hiccup. A pleasant look would cross her face as I changed her diaper and then she would startle. Was she afraid of the diaper change? Although that seemed like a small and not terribly alarming reaction, from experience I knew something wasn't right. So, after a couple weeks, I took action.

As a habit, I don't go out of my way to visit the pediatrician; there is a badge of honor worn by mothers of four or more children. We just don't have time to freak out over every earache. But funny hiccups were not in my medical repertoire, so I broke down and took Merritt to the doctor.

At the office visit the doctor decided Merritt should have an EEG just to rule out seizures. Everything else seemed quite normal for this darling ten-week-old little girl. She'd had her check-up two weeks before and been declared "perfect." We headed to Children's Hospital for the test.

I immediately disliked Children's Hospital. Sick kids, what is sadder than that? And how do you not stare? And then every kid you see walking around with an IV on wheels makes you think, "When is he going to die?" After making it through the maze of corridors and brown and orange elevators, we entered the neurology clinic and I was convinced we'd be leaving "The Realm of Pitiful Kids" within the hour.

Our sweet little peanut was wrapped up in a straitjacket. Like a mini psychopath she had to endure restraints while strangers drew black dots on her head. After all the dots were on her head, twenty-three electrodes were glued on with multi-colored wires running to a machine. These looked like the same kind of wires her older sister Paige made into bracelets at camp. The technicians made us leave the room. We stumbled back to the waiting area, to sit with all the sick kids and their parents. I wished I could just crawl in a hole. We didn't belong in this place.

After about an hour and a half the technician called us back to the testing room. There was a new lady in the room. She had a mellow funeral-director voice. Most people at Children's try to have that "oh-it-is-so-special-to-have-you-here" voice, so they don't scare the bajeebees out of the kids. But dimly lit room and this lady's pallor and low tone conjured up images of The Addams Family. If the setting alone wasn't enough to make me run, the words out of the Pediatric Neurologist's mouth, "seizure activity," had me one step closer to grabbing my baby and running to the elevator. Merritt would be admitted for more tests.

Merritt was ushered to different parts of the hospital for a five full days of tests. As I carried Merritt from test to test I was a mama monkey picking at the flakes of leftover glue on her precious head. Soon, surely, someone in this world-class children's hospital would walk in and give us an answer. Wouldn't they?

Incredibly, it would be six months before we would get a definitive answer. But we didn't need tests to tell us that Merritt wasn't developing. At seven months of age she was still at about the level of a normal three-month-old. She continued to have seizures; she was diagnosed as legally blind; she had almost no muscle tone. Our doctors had ruled out all muscular diseases and were starting to think her issues were metabolic. The word sounded like bubonic, a horrible plague from the Middle Ages.

I would learn that "metabolic" describes how nutrients are metabolized in the body - or, **how the cells get fed**. Merritt's doctor suspected a mitochondrial disease. **The mitochondria are little fish-type compartments in every cell that supply the cells with energy.** Energy was something Merritt definitely lacked. She slept at least eighteen hours a day, couldn't hold her head up, and had difficulty eating. We had no clue how to proceed.

Out of desperation, I asked the Doctor, "What would you do if this were your child?" He sent us to Atlanta.

There is nothing wrong with Atlanta. It's a great city. Unless you're going there to discover the potentially horrible fate of your eight-month-old baby. We made the best of our first night, enjoying some Mexican food and margaritas, while Merritt slept soundly in her infant carrier at our table.

We visited the doctor who was supposed to be the best in the field of mitochondrial diagnosis. A surgeon had to take a muscle biopsy from Merritt's thigh. It would be delivered to the specialist's lab where five thousand cells would be spun, separated and diagnosed. The whole process would take three months. What to do while waiting? The eternal question. I wondered how many margaritas it would take to keep me numb for three months.

After returning from Atlanta, Merritt was scheduled for another MRI. Some parents take their kids to Sears Photo Studio every couple months; we took our baby for brain pictures. Her first MRI showed that the myelin sheath that covers the brain was not developed. Without that sheath, Merritt's brain constantly misfired, causing the seizures.

Merritt's hour long MRI was on a Friday. Happy TGIF. Her doctor said he'd try to get back to us that day, but it may not be until after the weekend.

Sometimes you feel an event is going to be pivotal in your life even before you know the full spectrum of it. When the phone rang at 8:30 on that Friday night and caller ID popped up "PittChilHosp" I sensed I was entering "That Moment When Our World Would Change Forever."

The scan was carefully explained. Merritt's brain had decreased significantly since her last MRI, four months prior. With this information we knew the results from Georgia would not be encouraging. "Merritt has a degenerative disease," the doctor said solemnly. "And it is progressing fairly rapidly. She may live two years."

Degenerative. What does that mean? Digressing? Disintegrating? Disabled? I looked it up. Degenerate: deterioration of a tissue or an organ in which its function is diminished or its structure is impaired. Her brain was deteriorating. All the "d" words were bad.

I cried a lot. While sobbing on the phone with my sister and then my mom, I kept the wine flowing. But the next morning I not only woke up sullen but also hung over. Drinking, I realized, was not the best way to get through this.

13

So, to the laundry room I trudged. That space was mine for a reason. Since we first realized something was wrong with Merritt, I'd found myself more and more drawn to this unorthodox sanctuary that smelled of Tide and mildew. I went there to pray, mourn, cry and search.

As the Queen of Positive Attitudes, I had never faced a tragedy. In college I annoyed my roommate when I'd quote Robert Schuller's "Power of Positive Thinking." "If it's going to be, it's up to me." Nothing like a televangelist to get a good dose of PMI (positive mental attitude).

God and PMI had never let me down before. But before was different. Anything before that Friday night phone call was manageable. It was, basically, small stuff. This was big stuff and I needed bigger help than my storehouse of optimistic buzzwords.

Without a definite diagnosis we still weren't sure what we were dealing with. But, we knew Merritt would not be growing up.

We had three months to wait for the test results from Georgia: June, July, and August. During other summers, I planned outings with the kids, registered for camps, swam every day, packing the days full and letting the kids drop into bed, happily exhausted.

But this summer I didn't have it in me. Depressed and still trying to sort out my feelings, our summer, and my sunny personality, were overcast by Merritt's seizures.

Simplifying the summer actually taught me a lot about savoring. Holding Merritt, I would sit on the front porch bench and watch the kids play. I soaked up their laugher as they ran through the sprinkler and played freeze-tag. My children were old enough that they didn't need to be watched as they played outside, at least not closely, but I needed to absorb them that summer. While waiting for those test results I needed to rejoice in my precious children. If I was going to adapt to a child who wasn't going to be normal, I had to learn some really hard lessons.

"Horizon" popped up on the caller ID the first week of August. As soon as I saw the name of the Atlanta Lab, the joy of summer drained and dread poured into my veins. The test results were in. Would I like them "mailed or faxed?" a sweet Georgia voice asked.

"Hmmmm, should I agonize for an additional few days, or end the year-long torture?"

I couldn't look. Is this how people feel when they ask the ultrasound technician to seal the test results about the baby's sex because they aren't sure they want or need to know that bit of information quite yet? "When I'm six months along, then I'll need to know." Something within me wanted to postpone knowing the answer right that second. I didn't want to find out about the future of my baby's life on a hot August afternoon, staring down at a fax machine.

Soon, however, I couldn't stand the suspense. I flipped the papers over. I searched the 17-page document for the word: diagnosis. On the seventh page I found it. Leigh's Disease.

The air thickened and the tears started. Maybe I should have waited six more months, to postpone this sorrow. There are many mitochondrial defects and with some, a person can live an almost normal life. Although we didn't expect Merritt to have one of the best ones, we also didn't expect the worst. From the research I had done, I knew Leigh's was the scum of these disorders.

During those months of waiting I tried to prepare for the worst news. But there is no way to prepare for tragedy or to understand how it will permeate your pores. And of course I, the eternal optimist, thought we'd have better news to digest.

"Mom, why are you crying?" Paige, my oldest, asked as I threw the report on the kitchen table.

"We finally know what's wrong with Merritt. And I'm sad."

While trying to prepare for Merritt's diagnosis we had been very open with our older children about her "funny brain." We had described her as one of God's special babies.

Paige, in the comforting role of first born, said, "Mom, remember, Merritt is one of God's special babies."

Kids forget to brush their teeth and finish their math homework, but it is uncanny how they can remind you of the words of hope you've spoken to them. I needed reminding.

That night I tried to put up a good front. When sadness is thick, kids turn puppy-like. With an approaching thunderstorm, they seemed to circle around me, gently nudging and whining. They didn't know how to interpret the news, they only knew it was bad and wanted to feel the comfort of parental love. A nuzzle, some reassuring strokes. It took everything in me to put them to bed with the reassurance that God knew what He was doing.

After the children were in bed, I headed for the laundry room in search of peace. I moved slowly, postponing the moment when the laundry would be done, and I would need to put Merritt to bed with the knowledge that one day she wouldn't be with us.

For a whole year I had been planning for this time; how would I deal with the diagnosis? To my surprise I didn't need four glasses of wine. The worst part of Merritt's disease had been waiting for the results. Now we had them and to my surprise, there was peace in the finality. An inexplicable calm filled me.

We had a highly special needs child, who would most likely never develop beyond her current infantile level. Her cells would not be able to sustain her vital systems and she would eventually decline physically and have an early death. It wasn't the news I wanted, but it was in my basket to sort out.

What's a Mom to Do?

Hmm...not the news anyone wants. I knew at that moment I had to take control of at least one aspect of my daughter's life. Doctors were controlling a lot. I wanted to get in on that, I was the mom! Somewhere in all the discussion of my daughter's condition I latched on to one phrase: **Doesn't process food into energy**.

Food. I knew food. I loved food. I studied food in college. Before having kids, I sold imported foods to high-end restaurants. And besides just knowing food, I embraced an alternative eating style already. In Pittsburgh vegetarianism at that time was still thought of as odd. "What do you mean you don't eat meat? Don't you crave a burger?" was a line of questioning I often heard. But I had been vegetarian for a number of years and I realized I had a lot of energy. (Don't get scared...this isn't a book about becoming a vegetarian!)

To gain a bit of control I took over Merritt's diet. No more typical stuff. I was on a mission to feed her cells. If she couldn't process food properly, I would at least give her a fighting chance by giving her food that would be easy to convert. Mitochondrial disease is known as the disease of no energy. The United Mitochondrial Disease Foundation's slogan is "Hope. Energy. Life." I had to do something. Merritt was sleeping her life away. Merritt needed energy.

Since Merritt's diagnosis I have become an expert in ENERGY. Four kids in seven years, a special child and a crazy optimistic attitude have sustained me through the journey. And the changes I made in Merritt's diet have sustained her. At the time of writing this book, Merritt just turned twelve. She is severely disabled, infantile really. But she has never been hospitalized, never received a feeding tube, and doesn't get colds or ear infections or even fevers. The childhood illnesses that most kids deal with haven't been an issue for her. Her doctors are amazed.

Her neurologist told me, "Just keep doing what you're doing. We don't have time to study what you know, but it is working and I don't know another child like Merritt."

Merritt's middle name is Joy. When I named her, I had no clue that her purpose in life would be just that. She is a child who will never talk back, the police will never call me and tell me she's in trouble, and she eats everything I put in her mouth. People ask me if it is hard to have a child like that. I answer, "No, she is pure joy!"

The rest of this book will walk you through some of the lessons I have learned and inspire you to make changes so you gain energy in your life. No one wants to sleep through their days. I want you to wake up and go get your joy on!

Chapter 2

Eat Energy-Producing Foods

N

E

R

G

Y

A Lesson in Real

I met Charlotte, a holistic nutritionist, who I thought could help me with Merritt's diet. After a couple hours of consultation I left Charlotte's office with a juicer, a bag full of supplements and a pint-sized portion of hope. With newfound enthusiasm, I was going to feed my baby's cells. **I learned that 50% of our energy consumption each day goes to the process of digesting food and turning it into energy.**

Certain foods are harder to digest and even the way we eat foods put more of a drain on our bodies. Think about that food coma you're in every Thanksgiving afternoon. Your body is working hard, really hard to digest Grandma's sweet potatoes, a mountain of stuffing and the three "slivers" of pie that were part of your meal. And while you're digesting, your body is snoozing. So what foods should you eat for more energy?

I'm Heading to Whole Foods

The parking lots are crowded, the aisles are narrow and the food is organic. That's the image that may come to mind when I say "whole foods." But I'm not talking about the upscale grocery store where you can sip a wheat grass juice while buying gluten free pizza crust. For 500 generations, people grew what they ate. We have now had two generations that don't eat what they grow. We don't eat whole foods.

Whole foods are foods in their raw natural state. We've become so removed from this process that we consider a product like sun-dried tomato and basil crackers to be a real food. But if you were to read the ingredient list on that box, you would realize these crackers weren't grown on a vine, nor were any of their ingredients. When I say whole foods, **I mean real, as close to the form they are grown**. Think the opposite of Taco Bell's Doritos Locos Taco®. Really? What is that? Or how about a GoGurt®? A tube of what? A yogurt-type product. Instead, picture an apple. Can you see the tree it grows on? Now you've got it.

Whole real foods grow in the ground or sea or they had a mama or came from a mama with minimal to no processing. If there is an ingredient in your food that doesn't meet those two criteria, then it has been processed and isn't whole. If it isn't a name you recognize, then it isn't real. Whole, Real Foods. Remember it.

Your cells create energy when they are fed nutrients. The nutrients cells need to make energy are found in whole, real foods. Do you have any? Open up your fridge. We're going to go on a journey deep down between that rotten cucumber and the container with the left over bean burrito. The key to your energy levels and zest for life lies behind the refrigerator door.

Four Reasons Whole Foods Give You Energy

Okay. Is your fridge open? What do you see? Take a quick inventory. Fruits? Veggies? Whole foods? (If you're having any doubt about what whole, real foods are, refer to BONUS CHAPTER. Twenty of my top superfoods are listed there.) The list of reasons to eat these types of foods is long. But I'm going to break it down into four reasons whole, real foods give your cells what they need to make energy.

Reason Number One:

Whole Foods Give Us Plant-Based Chemicals

Whole, real foods give us polyphenols, flavonoids, and phytonutrients. These are all a bunch of words that mean a bit of the same thing. They are plant-based chemicals. I used this terminology one time and an audience member said, "I thought chemicals were bad to eat!" She was right about artificial, lab-produced chemicals. But I'm talking about the chemical compounds that make up food. Natural stuff.

Picture an orange. That is a pretty natural thing. Close your eyes. Think about what it smells like when you rip off a section of the skin. What does each segment feel like? What happens when you bite into a section? When you experience an orange, from the visual appeal to the smell and taste, you are experiencing its polyphenols, flavonoids, and phytonutrients. One hundred and six of these chemical compounds have been identified in an individual orange.

Scientists have discovered over 10,000 plant-based chemicals. They seem to know what about 1000 of them do at the cellular level BUT they speculate that there are as many as 40,000 undiscovered compounds. These compounds all affect the cell and the cell's functions. Some of the more commonly known phytonutrients include: lycopene, found in tomatoes, has demonstrated help in eye health, the resveratrol found in red wine is thought to help turn on anti-aging genes, and curcumin, found in the spice turmeric, has shown great anti-inflammatory properties.

Wow. Just think...a compound in the blackberry you ate this morning could unlock the secret to curing a degenerative disease like Parkinsons. The research in the field of food-based medicine is increasing at an exponential rate! While pharmaceutical companies spent the last fifty years developing compounds that help combat the symptoms of disease...Mother Nature has been quietly nurturing her own medicine cabinet of disease prevention.

So How Do All Those Plant-Based Chemicals Actually Give You Energy?

Your cells know what to do with them. Yep. Giving your cells these nutrients is like giving a puppy a bone. He knows just what to do with it. You don't need to give bone-chewing instructions to Bailey the dog. He just grabs the bone and is entertained for hours. Innate action. Cells take the compounds found in whole foods and use them to keep systems running at optimal levels. When your cells are given these phyto-boosters, they are equipped to perform. These plant-based chemicals are the superheroes of food. BAM, a virus is attacked. POW, inflammation is limited. OUCH, disease is prevented. When your body has what it needs to keep problems away, you then have more energy to study for an exam, power through a workout, or chase kids around the playground. **You have energy because your cells have fuel**.

When Merritt began eating a whole foods, plant-based diet, she woke up. She had been sleeping 18-20 hours a day. But with kale, blueberries and broccoli, she began to function. She started her day with a smoothie. And heck, if Merritt was getting energy from a smoothie, I figured it wouldn't hurt me to have one. For the last 11 years Merritt and I have started our day with a phytonutrient-packed smoothie. Morning is the best time to eat fruit and eating it alone without protein is the best way for it to digest and get the nutrients quickly to your cells. Here is our morning smoothie recipe:

Morning Wake-Up Smoothie

1 cup fresh pineapple

1/2 cup fresh or frozen blueberries

1/2 cup fresh or frozen raspberries

1 medium banana

1/4 cup mango fresh or frozen

2 TBS ground flax seed

2 TBS orange or pomegranate juice

Put all ingredients in a powerful blender. The Vitamix® works the best if you're using frozen fruit. If your blender is not that powerful, you may need to add more juice.

Although avoid adding too much, as juice is fruit without its fiber. Too much juice causes insulin to spike (we'll look at this when we discuss sugar!). This serves 2.

Reason Number Two:

Real, Whole Foods Give Us Antioxidants

If you haven't heard the term antioxidant, maybe you've been under a rock. Food manufacturers love to tout that their products contain antioxidants. But, it is in whole, real foods where you will actually find the most antioxidants. What are these miracles of nutrition? Antioxidants are molecules that fight free radicals. Ah, more superheroes.

Free radicals are the roaming by-products of normal metabolism and toxins in the body. So everyone has free radicals. But stress and poor diet increase the amount of free radicals. Free radicals are mainly oxygen molecules or atoms that are missing an electron. And they need that piece. There are only two ways the evil free radical can get its missing piece. It can steal it. Or it can be given one. What sounds better to you?

Have you ever played the game Jenga®? You build a tower out of blocks and then you slowly remove the pieces until the last possible piece that keeps the tower stable is finally removed. Tumble, crash. This is what free radicals do to cells. They steal pieces until the cell becomes unstable. Cells don't fall down, but they do die or they start making bad copies of themselves. Cells replicate by making copies. If you make a copy on a machine where someone has left a little white correction fluid on the glass, you know what type of copy you'll get. The smudge will appear on all fifty of the fliers you were going to hang to find your missing cat. Now your cat has a prominent black spot on his nose. If your cells get smudged by free radicals, they begin to make damaged copies. Before you know it, you have a problem. And that problem is called oxidative stress. Oxidative stress is this constant beating up of healthy cells by free radicals. And this is what leads to aging and disease. Not such good news.

But this is where whole, real foods save the day! Antioxidants in whole, real foods GIVE - yes, give - the missing pieces to the free radical. Pre-school teachers everywhere would be proud of all this nutrient sharing. When cells are whole and intact they can function at an optimal level and the risk of disease is dramatically reduced. And they can produce energy at the level that keeps you awake and thriving. So eating a wide variety of foods filled with antioxidants increases energy.

Foods have varying levels of antioxidants. The scale to measure antioxidant levels is called ORAC (oxygen radical absorbance capacity). But forget that. Really, the USDA has forgotten it. Don't get all excited about numbers and graphs that certain food products like to place on their labels touting their antioxidant properties. The USDA actually removed these numbers from their website because there was too much confusion over the values. All the numbers really did was to allow the blueberry juice people to give you a really cool graph on the bottle.

Generally, if a fruit or veggie is dark in color, it has a high level of antioxidants. So of course the berry family comes to mind. I take my kids black raspberry picking in the summer. Those stains on their hands and clothes are a pain, but that's the evidence of awesome antioxidants. Vegetables like kale and red peppers have high levels too. But that said, there is a really great antioxidant found in one of my favorite real, whole foods that isn't a really a vibrant color: the avocado. Avocados are an excellent source of glutathione, an important antioxidant that researchers say plays a role in preventing aging, cancer, and heart disease. And glutathione supports mitochondrial function which, remember, is where energy is produced.

Merritt has eaten a half an avocado every day for the last eleven years. The nutrients in avocado make it one of my favorite Super Foods (see more on Super Foods in my BONUS CHAPTER). For an awesome energy packed lunch, try this salad full of antioxidants:

Black Bean Avocado Salad

1 can organic black beans

1 avocado diced

1 cup kale, chopped fine

1/4 cup raw pepitas (pumpkin seeds)

1 cup cherry tomatoes, halved or whole

2 TBS olive oil

Juice of 1/2 lime

1/2 tsp cumin

Salt and pepper to taste

Combine everything in a bowl...easy, easy. Serves 2-4

Reason Number Three:

Whole, Real Foods Give Us Vitamins and Minerals

Vitamins and minerals are a key component to vitality. And, 90% of all Americans do not get the vitamins and minerals they need each day. Wow. Think about that number. Nine out of ten people walking around are deficient in components that help them thrive during the day. Imagine if 90% of Americans walked around without their cell phones! Teens everywhere would be lost and irritated when they couldn't update Twitter or post pictures. And most of us would miss appointments or miscommunicate all day long. **Without vitamins and minerals your cells are irritated and miscommunicating!**

Vitamins are found in living things, so we get vitamins from food that was alive. Or in the case of Vitamin D, we get the most usable form from the sun. Minerals come from dirt. Water washes over rocks and substances in the dirt, plants absorb the minerals or animals eat the plants that absorb the minerals, and we eat those plants or animals and receive the minerals. We can also supplement with vitamins and minerals, and that is discussed in Chapter 8.

Vitamins and minerals play roles in metabolism, cell growth and health, organ function, and maintenance. Without proper levels of vitamins we wouldn't be able to see in color, bones become brittle, blood doesn't clot when we're injured, hormones (including the ones that control sex drive!) become unregulated, the list goes on and on!

The best way to understand what happens when we're deficient in these vital nutrients is to visit the ER. Not literally, but join me as I relive a visit to the Emergency Room:

My eight-year-old daughter was streaking through the house like she was being chased by an ax murderer. High-pitched screams had been alerting me to some spirited play going on upstairs for the last few minutes. With four children in the house, high-pitched screams and loud noises are normal. I don't get too stressed out by the fun. But when eight-year-old Paige came flying through the kitchen, my ears perked up and I turned. As I turned, I saw her six-year-old brother JP in fast pursuit of his fleeing sister. Just then she threw open the door to the basement. Unfortunately she threw it open directly into JP's face. The doorknob caught his cheek, right at the bone beneath the eye. A high-pitched scream of another sort rang through the house. One look at the gash and I knew where we were going. My afternoon would be spent in the ER.

All three of us, Paige (along for sympathy and guilt), JP and I, crammed into one section of the revolving ER door. JP stood pathetically holding a droopy, wet washcloth to his cheek as I checked us in with the ER nurse. "Please go have a seat and we will call you when we're ready," she instructed. JP turned his eyes up to me and with a questioning look I could tell he wondered exactly what would happen to him behind the swinging doors.

We settled into the waiting room. The soda and candy machines were calling my kids' names, so I attempted to entertain them with a few rounds of "I Spy." After about 45 minutes of waiting, JP's wet wash cloth dropped to the floor, Paige was longingly eyeing the Reese's Cups®, and I had spied everything from what looked like a heart attack patient to unknown fluids on the floor. Everyone's patience was running out.

I asked Paige to sit still and I took JP by the hand back over to the nurse who had checked us in.

"Excuse me. Do you have any idea how much longer it might be until my son is seen?" I said in my politest don't-mean-to-bother-you-but-we're-tired-of-waiting voice.

The nurse looked us up and down, obviously trying to place us and the significance of our injury, "You should be happy you're waiting," she replied as I gripped JP's hand a little tighter, "you are not a very big emergency."

We slumped back to our chairs. We had just experienced the practice of triage. If you've never been to the ER you've at least probably seen one on TV. Triage is the practice of assessing the seriousness of an injury and assigning an order to which patients are treated. Some emergencies are just bigger than others. Heart attacks vs. flesh wounds – heart attack wins every time.

So what does all this ER stuff have to do with our cells and vitamins and minerals? Everyday your brain is playing triage nurse. Yep. Vitamins and minerals are needed by a lot of organs in your body. But remember, you and the majority of all people are not getting all the vitamins and minerals you need. So some part of you must figure out what is the most important or critical area that needs a nutrient. And once that is decided, every other organ sits and waits. Let's look a little closer at just one vitamin.

Let's pick on Vitamin D. Vitamin D is a very important vitamin. It is used by about 32 of your 76 organs. Well, you wake up one day and stay inside. The most usable form of Vitamin D comes from the sun. No sun for you today. You're studying, working or lying on the couch. As some of those organs start crying out for vitamin D, your body's triage nurse starts assessing the situation. "Hmm. Not enough D for the thyroid today, better not send it there. The liver needs it. The liver is a vital organ...can't live without a liver." That is the type of cellular communication happening inside you when you don't have enough of a particular nutrient to go around. No big deal, right? Thyroid can get by okay for today. An underachieving thyroid isn't going to kill you. Nope. But the thyroid does control your hormones. So maybe today you don't metabolize your food into energy well, you feel completely overwhelmed and stressed, you anger easily, you're tired, your digestion is off, you have no sex drive. Yep, the thyroid is just a little organ that isn't too important. Not.

The concept of triage nutrition makes a very clear point. **If you are not getting all the vitamins and minerals your body needs, your organs are not getting what they need.** You are deficient. You lose energy and the ability to function at your optimal levels.

To stay fully energetic you must get vitamins and minerals from real, whole foods.

One mineral that many people are deficient in is magnesium. Magnesium is known as a master mineral and is responsible for the activity of 300 metabolic processes. Some symptoms of low magnesium are: weakness, calcium deficiency, muscle cramps, anxiety, high blood pressure, poor memory, confusion and poor heart health. Doesn't sound like you can be terribly energetic and engaged when you're deficient in magnesium, does it?

A favorite source of magnesium for me is nuts and seeds. I'm a huge fan of keeping a container of sunflower seeds, pumpkins seeds and almonds mixed together. Pumpkin seeds are often sold as pepitas and are green. Buy seeds raw, not roasted, to get all the health benefits they offer. Other sources for magnesium: dark leafy greens, brown rice, bananas, and fish.

Reason Number Four:
Whole Real Foods Provide a Synergistic Balance of Nutrients

Remember in grade school when it was time for music class? The best day was when the music teacher got out the magical box of instruments. Generally a small riot broke out over the cymbals. The triangle was kind of cool, too. When everyone first got their instruments there was generally a cacophony of noise. No real music. But then the teacher put up a rudimentary chart that somehow you followed along to and before you knew it "Row, Row, Row Your Boat" never sounded more fluid. The instruments played together had a synergy.

The beauty of a symphony orchestra is magical, even more so than what is produced in first grade music class. If you have ever had the opportunity to listen to a professional orchestra live, you know that the balance of instruments gives a sound that is exhilarating and powerful. But before the conductor comes to the podium, those professional musicians warming up their instruments are not too different than the children with their triangles and cymbals. The synergy just isn't there until the conductor brings it all together. The pieces are operating independently.

When we eat a food in its whole, real form, we eat a synergistic balance of nutrients. A whole carrot is a symphony and your brain is conducting. Science knows how to break the nutrients down in a carrot. We can mimic the Vitamins A and C and even the beta-carotene found in a carrot. We can take a pill or powder and get those nutrients. The nutrients can play on their own. But science has proven that breaking foods into components does not lead to ultimate health. Your body needs food in its whole form, because your brain knows how to get the food broken down so all the parts are used. Remember, we still don't know what all those plant-based nutrients do. But the great conductor inside you does.

Ultimate energy comes when our cells receive all the components of a food. One of the most frequently asked questions I receive is, "Can't I just take some vitamins?" I will address this question in chapter 8, but for now, understand that we were made to live on food. Mostly plants and some animals in their whole, real form. These are the instruments your body understands and that science has yet to master.

Eat for Energy

Without the power of real, whole foods our cells don't receive what they need to thrive. Cells make compromised copies of themselves, systems are not fully supported to fight disease, aging occurs at a rapid rate and we lack energy! When bodies work hard, just

A Carrot Is A Carrot Muffins

1-1/2 cups whole wheat flour

1-1/2 cups shredded carrots

3/4 cup flaxseed meal

2 apples shredded, with peel on

3/4 cup oat bran

1 cup chopped walnuts

3/4 cup brown sugar

3/4 cup milk or almond milk

2 tsp baking soda

1/4 cup plain Greek yogurt

1 tsp baking powder

2 eggs

1/2 tsp salt

1 tsp vanilla2 tsp cinnamon

Mix together flour, flaxseed, oat bran, brown sugar, soda, powder, salt and cinnamon in a large bowl. Stir in carrots, apples and nuts. Combine milk, eggs, yogurt and vanilla in a small bowl. Pour liquid ingredients into dry. Stir just until moistened – do not over mix. Batter will be very thick. I use an ice cream scoop to put batter into greased muffin tins. Fill muffin tins 3/4 full. Bake 350 for 15-20 minutes. Yields 15 regular size muffins or 48 mini.

to function at a sub-optimal level, there is no energy left to live an engaged and vital life.

Your body needs fruits and vegetables, yet the majority of Americans get a scant portion of what they should be consuming of these foods. The majority of the country considers French fries a vegetable.

For optimal health and energy you should incorporate 7-10 servings of fruits and vegetables daily into your diet. Yes, you read that right. The five-a-day deal that has been pushed by the government funded education programs just isn't enough for cellular health and optimal energy. And think about it, if you're filling yourself with servings of whole, real fruits and vegetables, you're not filling yourself with Whoppers and KFC® Buckets.

You will learn more about what foods you should be eating in the BONUS CHAPTER – 20 Superfoods!

Kathy's Best-o Pesto

Summer isn't complete without a big bunch of basil turned into delicious pesto. Flavonoids in basil have been shown to protect cell structure of white blood cells. And anti-bacterial properties of herbs like basil, thyme and rosemary are present in the volatile oils in the plants' leaves.

It has taken me a few years to actually remember what I do when I make pesto. Usually I make it by feel. But I was teaching my daughter to make it one summer, and realized I better measure and record. Here is my best:

Kathy's Best-o Pesto
(*Continued*)

4 cups basil leaves

4 cloves garlic, smashed and roughly chopped

1/2 cup walnuts or pinenuts

1/2 cup extra virgin olive oil

1/2 cup parmesan cheese

1/2 cup water

1/2 tsp salt

1 TBS balsamic vinegar

Combine the basil and garlic in a food processor. Pulse for 2-3 seconds. Add the nuts and pulse a couple times. Add the remaining ingredients and process until smooth. Add more olive oil or water to make it your favorite consistency.

Chapter 3

E

Not Sugar And Caffeine

E

R

G

Y

Sugar Is Sweet and So Are You!

On Merritt's third birthday I decided to make a cake. In my previous before-all-healthy-food life, I was a wonderful baker. Butter, sugar, frostings, fillings...oh my. I did it up right when it came to baked goods. But the more I studied the effects of sugar on our cells, the less baking I did. But it was her birthday for goodness sakes! Merritt ate a plant-based, whole foods diet. She started her day with the smoothie mentioned in the last chapter, ate gluten-free cereal with avocados and vegetables for two lunches, and finished off her evening with a tofu, almond butter and kale puree. No cake. Kind of sad, right? That is how I was feeling on her third birthday. Surely this little girl who only ate pureed natural goodness deserved a bit of chocolate cake. (Let's be real for a minute; *I* wanted cake).

Pulling out my heavy stand mixer, I diligently measured and plopped sour cream and melted chocolate into the bowl. This chocolate cake was one of my favorites and I was going to give my child a treat. We all do that. Use food to love people. On my refrigerator I have a sticker that says, "Love People, Cook them Tasty Food." So all the pent up mom feelings of depriving my daughter of a sweet came out on her birthday. What resulted from my afternoon playing Cake Boss was a four layer, fudge-filled extravaganza. It was a labor of love and worthy of a role in a Food Network challenge. (I can't however tell the story of this cake without mentioning that we were dog sitting our neighbor's 100-pound Airedale and while the cake sat on the counter, he was able to take a bite out of one side! That side faced the back for pictures.)

As relatives arrived to celebrate our special little girl's milestone birthday (This was her third birthday and remember, she was only supposed to live to two!) I marveled at the spectacle of confection that was her birthday cake. After dinner and candles and the singing of *Happy Birthday*, I ceremoniously cut a tiny bite for Merritt. Merritt cannot chew but I was hopeful that she would enjoy tiny pieces of cake. Or at least the frosting. Oh, that frosting. An amazing, decadent fudge delight.

I swiped my finger through the frosting and although tempted to lick it off myself, I put it on Merritt's lips. Her tongue approached it tentatively. As she began to smack her lips, she did the most amazing thing. **She spit it out.** That child made the face that most toddlers make when they encounter lima beans! Her nose crinkled up and she tried everything to get the sweet substance out of her mouth. I felt a pain in my heart. Who spits out fudge frosting?! I decided not to attempt to force feed her cake and instead watched my other children devour their sister's cake.

Merritt was not accustomed to sweets. She did not eat any processed sugar and therefore did not like the taste. Unfortunately that is the reverse situation of nearly the entire US population. **We are addicted to sugar.**

In the 1970's when I was in grade school, the average American ate 20-30 pounds of added sugars a year. Fast forward to present day. If I was wheeling my grocery cart through the aisles of my mega-market and decided to fill it with the amount of sugar the average American eats today, I would be plopping in 27 five-pound bags. The average American consumes 135 pounds of added sugar per year.

That is a ton of sugar. Literally. A family of four would eat a TON of sugar in less than four years.

How did this happen? If you look at charts of sugar consumption over the decades, there is a major jump in the late 1970's to early 1980's. This is when the process to produce High Fructose Corn Syrup (HFCS) became streamlined and allowed manufacturers to use a cheap alternative to cane and beet sugar. Corn became the king of sugars. The phrase Supersize was coined. And our current epidemic of obesity and diabetes was born.

We use sugar not only for the taste, but we know that after we get a bit in our systems, we have some energy. That is a false energy. That is not our cells getting nutrients like phytonutrients, vitamins and minerals, but rather our cells our being filled, and most often over-filled, with a spike that causes us to have a sugar high.

"But sugar is natural!" I hear this all the time. At the end of a lecture I was giving on the *Five Nutritional Habits of Very Vital People*, a hand shot up from a man during the Q & A. It is always hard to hear that sugar isn't good for our cells. I get that. We all want chocolate cake. I happen to be the bearer of bad news about the ill effects of sugar on the cells. I'm an easy target during Q & A. I'm talking smack on your cake. So the man with his hand waving asks, well really *states*, "But we need glucose to make energy. Why would sugar be bad?" Ahh, the misinformation of nutrition. This keeps me busy.

The man asking the question used the term glucose. When foods in their whole, real form (mostly carbohydrates), break down, they turn into glucose. And glucose is used by the cells for energy. Broccoli breaks into glucose. But refined sugar is not glucose.

White table sugar starts as a natural, real whole food: corn, beets or sugar cane. When sugar cane or sugar beets or corn are refined, the good, natural plant components are stripped away. What is left is sucrose. It is converted very quickly into glucose, but this is not the form of sugar that cells are begging for. Cells want the form of sugar found in broccoli (and all complex carbohydrates). So while the man who posed the question was somewhat indignant, I stood firm. I explained that there are 17 different manufacturing and chemical processes that sugar cane goes through to wind up as white table sugar. **This product is not natural.** When sucrose is isolated through the manufacturing process, it creates issues with blood sugar, hormone balance, digestion and immune function. All the good things that come with natural sources of sugar are missing. Sorry Mr. Nice Man With The Question, sugar in the form found in your sugar jar is not necessary for cellular function and energy.

But Why Is Sugar So Bad?

When the subject of sugar comes up during my lectures, I might as well be the school principal telling the student body that the school year has been extended by a month. I see the looks. I hear the moans. Yes, they're audible. I've even had adults get out their phones and start playing Candy Crush®. People will do anything not to listen to the lady who is going to take away Oreos® and Frappucinos. But I'm tough. I have four kids. I understand the role of bad guy. But this information on sugar is vital not only to your energy levels, but also your longevity and general health. So I can't sugarcoat the news: sugar is really bad.

Number 1: Sugar Is Highly Caloric

Let's forget calories for a minute. I hate to look at calories. Who cares? Calories are just a measure of energy and everyone burns them differently. We all have different metabolic rates. But for the sake of discovering more about sugar, let's just say sugar is high in calories. If we don't burn enough energy we gain weight. This is a no brainer. Too much sugar = weight gain. This is a book about feeling vital and you are not living at full vitality if you are overweight. Done with that.

Number 2: Sugar Messes with Your Insulin Response

Sugar in the body looks a bit like having babies. Keep up with me here; I've had a lot of babies. When you have your first child, every noise from that child elicits instant attention. You run to the crying baby, perform a full body scan and fix any minute crooked blanket or chilled appendage. When baby number two comes into your family, your response time to a cry is a bit slower. You've been down the block. You know sometimes babies just cry. You move a bit more slowly towards the fussy offspring but you eventually fix any problems. Child number three is a different story. You've been sleep deprived for several years. You know these babies have triggers that go off at the slightest discomfort. You also know that you are worn out and you just might not respond as quickly as the baby demands. But the child will be okay and eventually you'll do your best to solve her problems.

Sugar is a baby. Sugar is constantly demanding the attention of your body. This attention comes in the form of insulin. (In my example, mom = insulin). Insulin is the first responder to the needs of sugar in the body. Insulin must be produced by the pancreas and sent out into the cells to balance blood sugar. When we're young and our cells and organs work well, our insulin response is quick and attentive. But over time, insulin just doesn't respond to the screaming cells. Your insulin response team is worn out. Too many middle-of-the-night Big Gulp® and Skittles® runs. First you may experience slowed insulin response or metabolic syndrome (baby number 2). But after enough episodes of over-consumption of sugar your body will drift into a pre-diabetic or diabetic state (baby number 3). Your body is worn out and no longer capable of keeping up with the demands of sugar in your cells. Insulin is not adequately produced. You crash and must begin to take insulin via medication or shots.

Nothing good comes from living in a diabetic state. Every function in your body is compromised. To reduce the risk of this situation you must begin to limit your consumption of sugar.

Number 3: Sugar Suppresses Immune Response

My daughter Paige was a freshman in college. As she phoned home during her first semester she said, "Mom, my roommate is always sick!" Of course my natural response was, "What does she eat?" Paige replied, "All she eats is sugar! All day, tons of junk!" It did not surprise me that she was sick. When levels of sugar in the cell are high, immune response is low. Our cells can only handle so much activity and add-on jobs.

White blood cells act as your body's defenders. But in order to defend and maintain order, white blood cells partner up with a big dose of Vitamin C. If the white blood cells don't have C, they don't defend well. Think of Vitamin C as the ammunition inside a tank. An armed tank can do a great deal of damage defending an area, but without ammunition, it be rendered useless in a dangerous situation. Sugar disarms white blood cells. White blood cells take in Vitamin C from the blood stream. But here comes the sugar problem. Pesky sugar has a similar chemical structure as Vitamin C. Those darn white blood cells must have misplaced their night vision goggles, because they take glucose into the cell instead of C. The white blood cell gets overloaded with glucose and never takes in the Vitamin C. If blood sugar rises to levels of only 120...which can be obtained with a soda and a couple cookies...the white blood cell's ability to absorb and destroy bacteria is reduced by 75%! It can take white blood cells four to six hours to return to active duty!

People who have a sugar habit often are down and out with every cold and virus that floats past their nose. A suppressed immune function does not lead to an energetic lifestyle.

Number 4: Sugar Messes with Digestion

Bullying is everywhere. We have been on a national campaign to reduce bullying on the playground and internet. We have decided that bullying is unacceptable and we're making strides to eliminate it. But what if I told you that every day sugar is the bully on the digestive playground? Yep. Stealing swings and calling names is truly child's play compared to the havoc that sugar causes to the entire digestive process.

As the number of grams of sugar rose in the American diet, the number of digestive aids did too. A sit-com does not come to a conclusion without viewers being subjected to at least one commercial for a pill to solve all forms of digestive discomfort. We've become a nation full of heartburn, gurgling intestines, and stomach upset. We're supposed to eat, digest and have energy. But if we don't digest our food well, our cells don't get what they need. Our undigested or poorly digested meals become calories and byproducts, not energy producing nutrients. And sugar is to blame.

What happens when you finish off that pint of Ben and Jerry's® or slurp down a Carmel Macchiato? Digestion happens. Or rather, it is supposed happen. **Remember, fifty percent of your energy every day goes to the process of digesting your food**. When I changed

Vitamin C Rich Fennel Salad with Oranges

Forget munching down on a bunch of supplements; why not pack a Vitamin C punch with this simple salad? Besides the C in oranges, fennel has anti-fungal and anti-bacterial properties.

1 fennel bulb sliced in very thin slices

1 orange peeled and cut into sections or sliced into rounds and broken apart

2 cups baby spinach leaves

1/2 cup chopped walnuts

Dressing:

1/2 cup olive oil

2 TBS orange juice

3 TBS white balsamic vinegar (or red wine vinegar but use a bit less)

1 tsp honey

1/2 tsp Dijon mustard

Combine all the salad ingredients in a large bowl.

Combine all dressing ingredients in a jar with a lid. Shake vigorously and dress salad. Serves 2-4

Merritt's diet, I looked for the most efficient way to feed her; a way that required her to use the least amount of energy to digest. Eliminating sugar was first on the list.

Food enters the stomach in a specific order and empties in an order. Simple sugars are broken down first because they require very little effort to digest. Liquid, simple sugars like those found in sodas, energy drinks and juice require almost no digestion and they break down very fast. These and other simple sugars, like candy, cookies and jelly donuts must be dealt with quickly, and blood sugar levels are affected by how much enters your blood stream at one time. This is when insulin is produced. Complex carbohydrates like your lentils and apples and cauliflower break down second. Fiber in these foods slows the rate of digestion and the release of insulin. Then the breakdown of proteins occurs, followed finally by fats. When we eat fat we feel fuller longer, because fat stays in the stomach longest.

Say you go to your favorite restaurant for dinner. You have a traditional American meal. Salad, steak, starch, vegetable and because you can never pass up a piece of cheesecake or bread pudding, you add that on at the end. You get home, crawl in bed and at 3:30 am, your tummy is not happy. You're wide awake and feeling like you have a rock in your stomach. You have created a digestive scenario that makes all those purple pill manufacturers very happy. You need a digestive aid.

But if you had just skipped dessert, or waited a couple hours, your distress would have been so much less. Sugar jumped into the digestive playground in the form of cookies-and-cream cheesecake and now you're hurting. Your digestive system needs to deal with the sugar found in the dessert first. But you ate it last. So that piece of tenderloin and risotto with wild mushrooms sits undigested for several hours while the sugar from the cheesecake is broken down. The rest of the food doesn't get to play.

With the increase of sugar in our diet, digestion of food has gone from 24 hours, start to finish, to upwards of 72 hours. We are not digesting our food well and it is clogging us up. Add lack of fiber to the increase of sugar and we have become a nation of irregularity and intestinal inflammation. Not a good thing when you're trying to live an energetic life. We do not need to pop pills to reduce acid in the stomach; we need to reduce sugar so acid is produced at the right levels to properly digest food. When we reduce sugar, especially after large meals, digestion improves and more nutrients are available to the cells. Get on the anti-bullying bandwagon and kick sugar off the playground.

Number 5: Sugar Is Addictive

It's been called more addictive than drugs. People joke about their sugar addiction because it isn't illegal and most of us eat it daily. But what is dangerous and keeps us from living an energetic life is the obsession with sugar and the effects that addiction has on our bodies. Some of the same brain receptors that illicit drugs attract, the ones that trigger pleasure, are also triggered by sugar. You know the feeling. You eat a fudge brownie and you feel your whole body go, "Ahhh." A pleasure receptor has been hit. When we get addicted to this feeling, we eat and eat and eat sugar. We think about our next sugary treat. We plan ways to get it. If we leave our goodie bags at home, we make sure to stop off for more.

Are you addicted to sugar? I like this test. Imagine you walked into your home to find that someone had baked fresh homemade cookies. You are not hungry, you've just finished lunch. Are you able to pass on the cookies? Can you think, "I'll have one later when I'm hungry," or maybe you just break off a piece and are content with the taste. You probably aren't addicted to sugar. But if you look at the cookies and eat several, fully knowing you aren't hungry, you may be addicted to the taste and feeling of sugar. If you eat candy without even enjoying, but you just need to have sweets, then you may be addicted.

Sugar addition is bad for a number of reasons stated earlier. But if I had to pick the one reason that will eventually cause you to live a low-energy life, it is the lack of nutrients available to your cells when you are addicted to sugar. If you eat sugar, you most likely are not eating nutrients. Your brain gets this. When you don't have adequate nutrients, all those vitamins, minerals and phytonutrients your cells need, then your brain signals you to eat more. Your brain knows you need some selenium (a trace mineral) today but it has none. You will continue to get hunger signals when you're strung out on sugar because you need nutrients. But we don't know what the brain is looking for so we just eat more cupcakes. Because gosh darn it, cupcakes are good. Tell that to your liver. Your liver wants nutrients, not cupcakes. So the addictive quality of sugar keeps you from fully feeding your cells, and that keeps you from living an energetic life.

So Can I Eat Any Sugar?

During my lectures, after I extol the negative effects of sugar, the audience looks disheartened. I know I'm taking away your cupcakes. But some good news is coming. Our bodies can handle some sugar. Studies conclude that most of us can handle 35-50 grams of added sugar a day. Come on, that's not bad! You can have a cupcake. Or you can have a Hershey's® Bar. That is the iconic symbol that I like people to associate with sugar. Everyone knows what a Hershey Bar looks like. And that confection has 22 grams of sugar. But if you stroll down the grocery aisle you'll see that a cup of yogurt usually has about the same amount. And a Frappucino from Starbucks® usually has double that number. The important thing here is to hold on to that number and use it as a guide. When you decide to have a margarita and you realize it has the same amount of sugar as three Hershey's bars, you may opt for a light beer. Sugar hides everywhere. Start to become aware of how much you're eating.

But for optimal health, most of your daily sugar should come in the form of fruit or should at least be eaten with some fiber. It is when we drink our sugar (sodas and juice) that the most damaging effects occur. That is when insulin spikes high and our body has to do a lot of extra work to get blood sugar leveled out. It's also a good idea to get some nutrients with your sugar so the whole cake isn't a waste to your body. Think of it this way: eating a peach pie made with local orchard peaches and a homemade pastry crust is more nutritionally beneficial to you than a peach-flavored slushie from the local convenience store. Not all sugar calories are equal.

The next question that arises is: "What about brown sugar or sugar in the raw or agave nectar?" Everyone wants to know how to get their sweet on. And unfortunately all of these forms of sugar are still seen by your cells as glucose. It is all sugar. "But wait, surely honey must be good," I hear next. Again, your cells see this as the same stuff, BUT there are a few phytochemicals and natural compounds that make it healthier. The closer a food is to its natural state the better it is for you. So that means raw honey has even more beneficial properties.

Stevia is the one natural sweetener I love. Native to Paraguay, it is an herb that is 200 times sweeter than sugar. Just a pinch is a perfect way to sweeten your coffee or tea and your body does not recognize it as sugar! So no insulin response and no caloric intake!

What About Splenda® and Artificial Sweeteners?

The next chapter will look very closely at artificial sweeteners. But tricking your body with chemicals isn't a good practice. And I will show you why this can rob you of energy, too!

Ultimate energy comes to you when your cells are getting what they need to fully function. Sugar robs your cells of their ability to perform many functions. Sugar taxes many systems in your body including your digestive, endocrine, and immune systems. If you want to live a fully engaged and energetic life, it is wise to disarm yourself from the dangerous grip that sugar may have over you.

Not Caffeine

You've been trying to stay awake at your desk all afternoon. You have no idea why putting your head on your papers is so tempting. But slowly you feel your head start to slump. And then, "whoosh!" you snap your head back. Your co-workers could have awarded you a perfect ten for that head bob. But you've already depleted your bag of emergency M&M's®. That sugar buzz wore off and now you're crashing again. Caffeine, yes! Caffeine might do the trick. So you head to find liquid energy.

Mmm. I love coffee. So there you go. I can't possibly beat up on something I enjoy so much, right? Ah, but I drink decaf. See, about twenty some years ago I realized I was addicted to caffeine. And it wasn't coffee. No, I had a little habit that nice healthy girls don't talk about...I drank diet soda. I woke up and after brushing my teeth I popped open a can of ice cold, caffeinated diet soda. And that bubbly, chemical-filled beverage helped me get through not just my morning, but my whole day. I had a three-a-day habit. I planned my day around my sodas. When I was in college I knew exactly which buildings had the soda machines with the coldest drinks. While working my first job in corporate banking I would stare at my watch until it finally said 2:30. That was the time I allowed myself soda number two. But babies change stuff.

Kathy's Double Chocolate
Nutrient Dense Brownies

Here is a recipe I developed after years of making a brownie that was full of sugar and no additional nutrients. Yes, it was a good brownie, but so is this. And with the addition of pumpkin and whole wheat flour, you get some nutrients and fiber which slow insulin response and feed cells.

6 oz bittersweet chocolate, coarsely chopped

4 large eggs

2 TBS butter

3/4 cup brown sugar

1/2 cup pureed butternut squash, pumpkin or sweet potatoes

2/3 cup whole wheat flour

1/2 cup low-fat plain greek yogurt

1/2 cup Dutch processed cocoa powder

2 tsp vanilla

1/4 tsp salt

1/2 tsp baking soda

Melt the chocolate with the butter in microwave on medium power for 1 minute. Stir and repeat at 30-second intervals until melted. Whisk the flour, cocoa, salt and baking soda in a medium bowl. In a larger bowl, mix the eggs and brown sugar and squash until smooth, then add the yogurt and vanilla and mix. Whisk in the melted chocolate mixture until blended. Add the dry ingredients and mix just until moistened. Add the chocolate chips. Spread the batter in a 9 x 13 greased pan. Bake at 325 for 18 – 20 minutes.

When I was beginning to think about starting a family, I took a serious look at my diet. I did so many things right, yet here I was guzzling down chemicals and caffeine all day long. I knew I was addicted and I didn't like that habit. It had gone on for almost 15 years!

But I was weak. How could I stop something that made me feel so good? And my guess is many of you with either a sugar or caffeine habit feel the same way. And why stop? What could be wrong with it? Caffeine is natural, right? Hmm. I've heard that before.

It was the flu. A nasty lie-in-bed-for-two-days type of stomach flu convinced me to kick the habit. I had already gone three days without a diet soda. I was thinking of getting pregnant in the next few months. No better time than the present. Cold turkey worked for me. I missed my caffeine fix, but I was determined, so I adjusted.

What is caffeine and why are we so addicted? And ultimately, should we care? Ninety percent of Americans use caffeine. Funny, that is the same percentage of people who lack proper daily nutrients. We don't know how to get our vitamins and minerals but we sure know how to line up at Dunkin Donuts® and Starbucks for a shot of instant energy. But is it energy? And if it does give us energy, what is the point of eating leafy greens?

Caffeine Is a Con Artist

I am highly intrigued by the world of forgery. Art forgery is my favorite genre of deception. Over the course of history, great artists have been mimicked for profit. One of the reasons there were so many Rembrandt paintings in the past, over 1,000 of them at one point, is that every painting which looked ever so slightly like a Rembrandt would be signed by forgers. Now there are only about 250 signed, authentic Rembrandts. With the onslaught of forensic methods, a forger is easily foiled by infrared technologies and x-ray photography. Our bodies are not immune to forgery. And it is up to our brain to figure out the deception. Caffeine is the great con artist of energy.

In order to understand what caffeine is forging we must understand how energy is actually created and the role your brain plays. Hold on, here comes your human physiology lesson.

When a cell breaks down food the end product is called ATP, or Adenosine Triphosphate. ATP is the energy currency for life. It is stored in every cell. ATP is a big deal. It is synthesized in the mitochondria of the cell. (Remember, my daughter Merritt has a problem with the mitochondria in every cell in her body. Mitochondrial disease is known as the disease of no energy. Merritt is really good at low energy.) We get energy from ATP when one or more of its Triphosphates break away from the Adenosine. When all the phosphates are broken from the Adenosine, then it's time for your body to take a break. You have no more usable energy. You are now out of steam, your head is slumping ever closer to your desk. And your Adenosine is looking for a place to recover. Adenosine heads to receptors in the brain which then send a signal, "Hey, you're tired. Take a nap."

As your head is about to touch down, you suddenly remember the wonders of caffeine. And thus the greatest forgery of the century begins. **Caffeine's structure mimics Adenosine.** It signs its signature and hops right into those brain receptors, tricking your brain and you into a false sense of energy. And caffeine is such a good forger, it can take your brain four to six hours to figure out you have no real ATP in your cells. This is a sham that we have embraced with great enthusiasm. And museum directors are not around to authenticate our choices.

But is caffeine bad? It is a natural compound found in natural products. Look at coffee. It is a bean. Coffee has over 1000 different plant-based chemicals that are being studied for their effects on everything from Alzheimer's to weight loss. You can't get much more natural than a bean, or tea leaves, or cocoa pods. They all have caffeine. But the problem with caffeine is the form in which we take it.

If we all drank unsweetened Yerba Mate tea, a tea made from the bark of a tree that is high in caffeine, I may not even be talking about the ill effects of caffeine. But we have Five Hour Energy® drinks, teens dying from caffeine overdoses, and hazelnut-flavored lattes, so we have to address the hazards of caffeine.

The catalyst by which the caffeine is delivered is as important as the caffeine. Because I have a daughter in college I'm privy to some habits of young adults. While visiting with her on campus I witnessed a drink that made me cringe. Dubbed "The Trashcan," four or five bottles of different liquors were dumped upside down into a large plastic cup. The bartender seemed to count to three and then topped the concoction off with a squirt from the soda hose, possibly Mountain Dew® or Sprite®. The final crescendo came with a can of Red Bull® energy drink dumped upside down into the whole thing. And the point of the added shot of caffeine? You can stay awake longer to drink more, I presume.

Okay this may not be how you get your caffeine. Maybe you're just a morning coffee person. That's cool. I'm a morning coffee person, but again I drink decaf. After my addiction in my teens and twenties, I knew I didn't like that feeling. But if you do drink coffee, form is important. A large majority of Americans dump stuff in their mug. Sugar, artificial sweeteners and, my least favorite coffee additive, artificially flavored, non-dairy creamers, are all added to the morning mug as we attempt to become a part of the living world. In the next chapter I'll address the dangers behind these artificial foods, but suffice it to say, caffeine - like anything else - is best in the form closest to nature. Hazelnut non-dairy, non-fat, no sugar creamer is not too close to nature. If you want coffee, look for high quality beans, organic and fair trade are good, and just stick to coffee. Tea could be considered a better source of caffeine because of the plant based chemicals that have some healthful benefits. Green teas are better than black and again, unadorned is better than adding stuff to it.

If you choose to use caffeine, be wary of anything that uses the term "Energy" in its name. The type of energy that your cells produce comes from real, whole foods. Anything else is stimulants, sugar, artificial sweetener, flavorings and herbal blends that can be dangerous when combined. In 2012 there were over 20,000 caffeine related Emergency Room visits. Although it is natural, like any natural substance that is mixed with chemicals or alcohol, it can become dangerous. Real energy for your cells does not come from caffeine. Caffeine is not inherently dangerous to the body when it is in a very natural form. But it can become dangerous, even life-threatening, if it is over-consumed or combined with other stimulants or chemicals. To wake up in the morning and feel vital, you must feed your cells what they need.

Mocha Almond Cooler

My issue…I love the flavor of coffee. So I'm always looking for ways to get that flavor while avoiding caffeine and even too much coffee. Try this summer cooler. It gives the coffee flavor with added nutrients from the almond milk and dark unsweetened cocoa.

1 cup almond milk, unsweetened

1 cup very strong COLD decaf (or caffeinate if you must) coffee

1 TBS unsweetened cocoa powder

Stevia to sweeten

1 cup ice

Combine all the ingredients in a powerful blender. Puree until it looks like something you would buy at Starbucks. Serves 2.

Chapter 4

E

N

Eliminate Fake Food

R

G

Y

What Part of the Cow Is the Nugget From?

Sometimes things just sound wrong. My kids are pretty wise, and I must admit a bit food savvy, well...because I sort of did that to them. So a certain pride overwhelmed me a few years ago when Graham arrived home from fourth grade waving the lunch menu in his hand. "Mom, you are not going to believe what is on the lunch menu! Beef Nuggets!" I looked at him in utter disbelief. Really? This just sounded wrong and even my ten year old knew it. What could it possibly be? How was it made? Too many questions surrounded the menu option, but we didn't really care. Graham always packed his lunch.

What have we done to food? We've commercialized it, chemically enhanced it, genetically changed it, and taken the essence of whole, real food and demoralized it. Yeah, yeah, I know I'm on a soapbox. But I don't get it. Why are my children offered chemical-filled lunches when I had lunch ladies in hair nets arriving to school early to *make* food? Not open boxes and reheat stuff, but actually cook a school lunch. You know in France they still do this? Cook lunch. Novel concept.

Chicken Tenders with Parmesan and Herbs

The nugget is iconic. That is sort of sad. When I grew up a "nugget" meant gold and that meant you were rich! We have robbed our kids of a lot of nutrients by making the nugget one of the most recognizable foods. (And hardly any kids can recognize a turnip…I know, I've been in the classrooms with one!) But don't be disheartened. If your children or even you crave a nugget, make one that is delicious and nutritious! These are always a hit with my kids. And I once made them for 100 teens with only compliments and clean plates!

For bread crumb mixture:

1 cup whole wheat breadcrumbs (see note on how to make)

1/4 cup ground flax seeds

1/4 cup parmesan cheese

1 tsp Italian seasoning

1/2 tsp garlic powder

1/4 tsp salt

2-3 boneless chicken breasts/or a pound of chicken tenders

2 free-range chicken eggs

Preheat oven to 400 degrees. Coat a cookie sheet with non-stick cooking spray or a light coating of vegetable oil. Combine all the ingredients for the breadcrumb mixture in a shallow bowl. Cut chicken breasts into strips. In a separate shallow bowl whisk the eggs. Dip a piece of chicken

Chicken Tenders with Parmesan and Herbs

(*Continued*)

into the eggs, then into the breadcrumb mixture to coat. Place on prepared cookie sheet. Continue to dip the remaining pieces of chicken in the same manner. Place the cookie sheet on the bottom shelf of the preheated oven for 8 minutes. Using tongs, flip each piece of chicken over. The side that was down should be a bit brown and crispy. Put chicken back in the oven for 5 – 7 minutes until the second side is crispy. Serves 4-6.

Note: Whole wheat breadcrumbs can be made out of lightly toasted whole wheat bread or bread left out overnight to dry out a bit. Whirl the dry bread in a food processor or blender. Alternatively, whole wheat crackers can be used for a different flavor.

Would Grandma Eat It?

"What happened to our sense of eating that made us turn food into a product your great-grandmother wouldn't recognize?" That statement is directly from Michael Pollan, author and advocate of eating food in its whole real state. I mean honestly, could you imagine your great-grandmother eating a beef nugget? For 500 generations we grew the food we ate. For the last several generations we have become detached from our food supply. When we detach, we lose sight of what we're eating. If we want to have an energetic life, we must understand what we're putting in our bodies. What are we REALLY giving our cells to work with?

When I talk about the alteration of our food supply I like to start with a box of unassuming sun dried tomato flavored wheat crackers. That sounds kind of healthy, right? Tomatoes, wheat, not fried like a potato chip. It must be okay. But when the box is flipped over a host of fakeness is revealed. **When I say fake food I am addressing anything that is a chemical, additive, coloring, or processed ingredient**. In a box of presumably healthy crackers, you will find: three different artificial colorings, hydrogenated fats, and flavorings from the glutamate family. And if you don't know what that stuff does to your energy level, hold on, we're about to enter the underbelly of fake food.

Get the Food to the People and Give Them What Tastes Good

It's all about taste. No wait, it's all about money. The food industry is an industry. They exist to make money. Don't believe it? Ask their boards of directors what their mission is. Pay the shareholders, make a profit, and grow bigger to make more money. The way that food manufactures sell more food is to make a product consumers want to eat. Most consumers want food that tastes good, right? My kids would argue that sometimes I purposely look for food that tastes bad, but our opinion on the flavor of lentils varies greatly. For the most part, tasty food sells better.

In order to make food tastier, the food industry has at its disposal an arsenal of over 14,000 different additives. These additives make food last longer, taste better and look more appealing. And we gobble it up. I like to pick on Doritos®. They're iconic and everyone knows what nacho cheese flavored Doritos tastes like. And now with the fabulous collaboration with Taco Bell, one can have a taco made in a Doritos flavored shell. When I teach classes to children, I ask one brave child to come up in the front of the assembly and read the ingredient label on the back of the Doritos bag. They get corn right but when they get down the list, most of the ingredients become difficult to pronounce. It turns out a bag of Doritos is approximately 30% chemicals. Fake.

What are these fake foods and where do they come from? Entire books have been written on the subject and it is fascinating. But for the sake of our quest for more energy, I'm just going to touch on a few of the big players. These guys don't play fair when it comes to cellular health.

The Biggest Players in the Fake Food Round Up

The story of one of the grand daddies of food chemicals takes us back to World War II. When our troops returned from overseas there was talk about the better tasting rations that the Japanese possessed. Our government looked into the ingredients in those rations to see exactly why our troops began to complain about their own dull rations. Glutamate was the key.

Does that ring a bell? What about MSG? Ever hear of that? **Monosodium Glutamate** or MSG is just one of the many glutamates that are used to enhance the flavor of food. Glutamates are derived from seaweed; hence they can all be called natural. But what happens in the process to convert seaweed into glutamates is anything but natural. Keep in mind heroin is derived from poppies, so it is also natural. But when natural ingredients are synthesized into highly concentrated forms, they can become dangerous, even toxic. MSG has been labeled an excitotoxin by Dr. Russell Blaylock, MD. As a brain surgeon, Dr. Blaylock was becoming more and more concerned with the disease and damage found in younger patients' brains. He gave up his surgical practice to study the effects of this dangerous class of food additives. In his book, *Excitotoxins: The Taste that Kills*, Blaylock references his research that concludes that glutamates as well as aspartame can excite neurons in the brain causing cellular death. And get this: if the cells don't die right away, there is evidence of faulty cells accumulating over a lifetime until they trigger neurodegenerative disease. Not a fun or tasty alternative when you think of the consequences.

So you want to avoid MSG, right? You're going to do what any smart consumer would do; you're going to read the label. Your can of chicken noodle soup clearly states: NO MSG. This is good. But because MSG is "natural," food-labeling laws do not require it to be listed. Look a little more closely at the label, does it say, "Natural Flavorings"? This is code for MSG. Or how about autolyzed yeast extract? Yep, this also always contains MSG.

Many people first became aware of MSG because of something dubbed, "The Chinese Restaurant Syndrome." After eating a meal at a Chinese restaurant, many people noticed they got a headache or felt dizzy. Research went on to show that many Chinese restaurants have adopted the habit of sprinkling their food with powdered MSG. MSG increases the savory flavor of food. Skip the restaurant. Make your own Chinese!

Wow, That's Bright

I'm going to take you on a trip to Spain to tell you about the second big food additive we all take for granted. This one is in so many foods that unless you're aware of it and the negative effects it has on your cells you probably consume it every day. So let's go to Spain.

My daughter, Paige, went to Spain while she was in high school. Because she was privy to her mother's mild obsession with pure food, she was aware of some significant differences. I had very little contact with her as she was busy touring, but I was thrilled when I received a

Sesame Green Veggie Stir Fry

While colorful veggie dishes look vibrant, I like the looks of this all green dish when it's presented as a side or even as a main course. Add tofu or edamame for protein and you have a wonderful vegetarian dinner.

2 tsp dark sesame oil

2 TBS coconut oil or peanut oil

2 cups broccoli florets

2 green onions, sliced on diagonal about ½ inch long

2 cup snow peas, sliced on diagonal in ½

3 cups bok choy, chopped into 1 inch pieces

1/2 cup vegetable broth

2 tsp cornstarch

1 TBS soy sauce

1/2 tsp ground ginger

1/2 tsp red pepper flakes (optional if you like spice)

Heat a large sauté pan or wok over medium high heat. Add the coconut oil. Add the broccoli and onions. Cook for 3 minutes, stirring constantly. Add the sesame oil then the bok choy and snow peas. Sauté an additional 3 minutes or until vegetables are bright and still a bit crisp. Combine the stock, cornstarch, soy sauce and ginger in a small bowl. Add to the vegetables and cook 2-3 minutes until sauce is shiny. Serves 2-4.

Facebook message one afternoon. All it said was, "The gum has no color." And I knew exactly what she meant. European countries don't use nearly the amount of artificial colors in their food as we do in the U.S. And that goes for gum too. Face it; if you're chewing florescent green gum, some of that color is ending up in your cells. And what is so bad about blue sports drink or orange macaroni and cheese? Coal tar and petroleum sort of sum it up for me.

Yes, the list of food colorings that you see on the back of nearly every box, can and jar (unless it is organic or your aunt canned it) are derived from coal tar and petroleum. I like to hold up a vibrant blue bottle of Gatorade® when I talk about food dyes. The only place you will ever find a color that vibrant in nature is on a tropical fish. Our food is not meant to be neon. But it sells better when it is color enhanced. Kids like it bright. Studies have been done that have people eating with dimmed lights. When the lights came on and they saw that the food is actually all grey, many of them became ill. Color and smell are part of the tasting process of eating. But these unnatural colors are damaging cells.

Originally there were over 200 approved food dyes. But over half of those were removed from use by the FDA or withdrawn from the industry. Links to liver disease, ADHD and even cancer have had the FDA recalling color additives for years. In 1973 the FDA banned Violet No. 1 because it was found to be a carcinogenic. For the previous two decades this dye had been used to stamp all meat sold in the United States as Prime, Choice or USDA. And we still have plenty to worry about when it comes to color additives.

The harmful effects of artificial colors in food are difficult to determine. Because these chemicals are used in combination with other chemicals, it is hard to pinpoint how and when disease or cellular damage occurs. But it does occur. Just ask any elementary school

Colorful Yogurt Without the Color

Much of the yogurt we consume in this country is artificially colored and sweetened. And if it is made to appeal to kids, you can pretty much guarantee it has a few! But it is so easy to flavor your own yogurt. The juice from the frozen berries makes the yogurt a naturally vibrant color. Get creative and get the kids involved!

1 16 oz. container unflavored Greek yogurt

1 cup frozen raspberries or blueberries, slightly thawed

1 tiny pinch of stevia

Mix all the ingredients together. Serves 2-4

teacher how her students behave after being given birthday snacks laced with numerous food dyes. The medical journal, *Archives of Disease in Childhood,* shared a study in 2004 in which four hundred children were tested for the effects of food additives on their behavior. The study showed "a substantial effect" of these additives on hyperactivity and behavioral problems. Many children are at a learning disadvantage with their morning bowl of cereal.

Not So Sweet

Okay. Now just a bit more bad news on the fake food front and then I promise we'll get to how all this ties your lazy butt to the sofa for the afternoon. The last fake food culprit that may be robbing you of energy comes in those ever-present yellow, pink and blue packets. Yep, we have to look at the dangers of artificial sweeteners.

My grandfather used to have a lazy Susan on his table. To entertain ourselves as the adults sat talking, my brother and I would tempt each other to spin it, without getting noticed or yelled at. The lazy Susan held the salt and pepper, a yellow plastic container filled with paper napkins and Grandpa's bottle of Sweet-n-Low. In the 1970's it was common to have a bottle of liquid saccharin sitting on the table. And we never gave it a second thought as Grandpa liberally poured the sweetener into his coffee.

Ahh, but a second thought is exactly what everyone should do when considering artificial sweeteners. Here is a brief history of the most significant players in the dangerous world of "Sugar-Free."

The saccharin that my grandfather used was the first artificial sweetener introduced. It was derived by researchers at John Hopkins in 1879, from a chemical called toluene, which comes from crude oil. It was never adequately tested before it came on the market for human consumption. In its long history it has been pulled off the market three separate times! Today its use is limited but it is still found in some prod-ucts, including drinks where it is often used as a blend with other sweeteners. It has been proven to cause cancer in lab animals.

Aspartame (NutraSweet® and Equal®) was my sweetener of choice all those years when I was addicted to diet soda. When the cola companies moved from saccharin to aspartame, much rejoicing was done by those of us with a habit. It had a more sugar-like taste and less after-taste. Yes, another food-chemical success story. Or not.

The G.D. Searle Company discovered the sweet substance later called Aspartame as they were trying to create a drug to treat ulcers. While trying to get FDA approval as early as 1973, the company submitted over 100 studies to verify the safety of the products. The FDA found the studies flawed and turned down Searle's request.

The role of the FDA is not to test the safety of products. Their role is to study the data that companies submit. Drug and chemical companies must produce their own studies and data. A few years ago while sitting around having some drinks, a friend who worked for a major drug manufacturer confirmed what I felt in my gut must be true. While discussing the role of the FDA, I asked him if he felt that his company's data submitted to the FDA was unflawed. He said, "About 80% of it is." Wow. I was shocked how easily that admission came out of him. Then he added, "I could get fired for what I just said." The topic of FDA approval is one that I have very strong feelings about. The very best book I've read on this subject is *The Hundred Year Lie* by Randall Fitzgerald. It is an amazing history of our flawed food supply and the agency that regulates it.

But, let's get back to our friends trying desperately to sweeten their soda and yogurt. After the failed attempt to get their product on the market, Searle committed even more resources to the approval. And then in 1977 Donald Rumsfeld became CEO of Searle. In 1981 he made a commitment to get Aspartame approved. Rumsfeld was on President Ronald Reagan's transition team. On January 21, 1981, the day after Ronald Reagan's inauguration, Reagan issued an executive order eliminating the FDA commissioners' authority to take action and Searle re-applied to the FDA for approval to use aspartame as a food sweetener. A few months later, aspartame was being added to my diet soda. The process by which this product became part of our food supply reeks of money and corruption. But that isn't the worst part.

The documented health effects of aspartame are the really tragic part of the story. The FDA receives more reports on adverse effects of aspartame than all other food products combined. Eighty percent of all complaints to the FDA involve aspartame. Amazingly, the FDA's own toxicologist, Dr. Adrian Gross, revealed to Congress that without a shadow of a doubt, aspartame can cause brain tumors and brain cancer. Research reveals that aspartame causes headache, memory loss, seizures, vision loss, coma and cancer. It can also worsen the symptoms of diseases and conditions like, MS, lupus, ADD, diabetes, Alzheimer's, fibromyalgia, chronic fatigue and depression. Umm, none of those diseases include heightened degrees of energy in their list of symptoms. Ultimate energy does not come from consuming this artificial sweetener!

But as much as we had a love affair with aspartame, we were easily wowed by the next sweet sham. Sucralose. Sucralose, most often known as Splenda®, is the nation's number one selling artificial sweetener. It is found in over 5000 products and is the primary sweetener in low carb foods, drinks and gum. In 1975 a graduate student at Queen Elizabeth College in London was trying to create a new insecticide - bug killer, that is. By slowing dropping highly poisonous sulfuryl chloride into a sugar solution the latest sweetener was born. Sucalose was denied approval by the FDA for eleven years (1987-1998). The other major players in the artificial sweetener world supposedly kept it out by wielding political power at the FDA. But then more games began.

In 1998 Monsanto wanted approval of its more intense, commercial-version of aspartame called neotame. At the same time they applied for approval, the FDA approved Sucralose. McNeil, the company behind Sucralose, was actually surprised and had to scramble to get factories ready. No documented data is available as to what actually took place for the FDA to suddenly approve both sweeteners at approximately the same time. But to this day, critics believe that the number of studies done on sucralose were not nearly sufficient to prove that sucralose does not have long term effects on human health. Some of these effects include: allergic reactions, blurred vision, gastrointestinal problems, seizures, dizziness, migraines and diarrhea.

And now, the ultimate blow to the sweetener is coming from some of those it was intended to help. Because the molecules in sucralose are not recognized by the body, they are not metabolized by the body. Or that is the thought. But studies are showing that in some people, anywhere between 15 and 40% of the sucralose is metabolized! So diabetics who use sucralose may actually be seeing a rise in their insulin levels. And something that affects even more of us, that unmetabolized chemical is turning up in our water supply.

When chemicals clog your system all the organs that keep your body clean work harder. Your liver is the key player here. And it works a lot like the filter in your furnace. Have you ever pulled out the filter or seen it when the furnace guy brings it to you and shows you a bunch of gunk and says, "Looks like you need a new filter"? Your liver is your body's main filter. The primary way in which your body expels toxins is via the liver. It detoxifies and cleanses your body by continuously filtering the blood that contains poisons that have entered through the digestive tract, the skin, and the respiratory system. So, it only makes sense that if your liver is working overtime to detox the chemicals you just threw in from your Doritos, Diet Coke®, and Skittles®, you're going to get tired. Your body works. Your organs do their jobs. But just like you, when you start piling on the exams, deadlines, extreme workouts, stress; you feel overloaded. And when your liver becomes overworked as a result of stress or excessive exposure to toxins, your entire system can be thrown off balance, and your health severely compromised. And guess what? You've got no energy.

Eating fake food is an energy buster. Not only are you not feeding your cells the nutrients they need, you're making certain organs work harder to clean out the junk. And if you haven't gotten the nutrients those organs need to work, they don't work as efficiently. The liver starts cleaning like a teenager, and trust me, that isn't well. When you do not filter chemicals out of your body and your liver clogs you set yourself up for disease. The bowl of neon orange cheese puffs seems like a good idea. They are a crunchy party in your mouth. But nothing good comes from the onslaught of damage these nutrient-deficient foods cause. Fake foods do not help you live a vital or energetic life.

Chapter 5

E

N

E

Reduce Stress

G

Y

Stress? Who Doesn't Have a Little?

Of course we all have stress. Even the most zen-like people I know are not immune to it. One bad day with a significant other, boss or kid and we all feel it. It doesn't take rush hour traffic or deadlines to make our body react to stress. A defiant teen walking out the door with a tiny skirt and a huge attitude is enough to escalate stress for the rest of the day. But how could stress possibly affect our energy levels? It is that rush of adrenalin that half of us have come to rely on to get through the day. Well, that and caffeine, right? Wrong.

Stress is *your body's response to a dangerous or life-threatening situation.* The life-threatening situation is supposed to be famine or physical threat – a bear chasing you. Not traffic or taxes. If you want to stay vital and stop living like a bear is chasing you, you must learn reduce stress. And I know a little bit about what it feels like to have a bear in pursuit.

The Bear Behind Me

The mountains of northern California's Sierra Nevada Range rose before us as we drew closer to Yosemite National Park. The blueberry pancakes we'd had for breakfast had fueled us for this long day of travel. And although I was uncomfortably full, I knew that I would burn mega-calories during the day ahead. We were trekking about ten miles that day, with heavy backpacks.

Before I had children I embarked on a two month Western odyssey with my former husband, John. We had a great plan to spend two months in the West before we started a family. Yosemite was on our list of must-stops. But not the valley. Oh no. Everyone goes to the valley. In our pursuit to shun crowds, we would head to the northern tip of the park and take two days to backpack down to the valley. We would have to earn those breathtaking sites in the heavily populated Yosemite Valley. We would have to hike past Half Dome before we could view it from below.

As we headed to the ranger's office I inhaled deeply the scent of pine that was thick in the air. No stress here. Until the ranger told us bears were all over our designated hiking route and we had to travel with a bear-proof canister for our food. John gleefully added, "I hope we see a bear." We had been through Wyoming, Montana, Idaho, Oregon and part of California without a single bear sighting. John felt a bear viewing was a rite of passage for this adventure. Two months without a bear encounter was like fishing and not catching. He was enraged when the active senior's group stepped off the red buses in Glacier National Park, giddy with pride at their bear sighting. They saw it out the climate-controlled bus window with their polarized prescription lenses – it shouldn't count. But we were slugging packs all over the west, without so much as a bear poop sighting. Secretly I was fine with it.

Half Dome, the sheer granite face that Ansel Adams made famous in his black and white photographs, was the incredible backdrop of our campsite. Fully aware bears were lurking in this highly traveled section of the park, we dutifully crammed anything that could be eaten into our bear-proof canister. "Would a bear drink contact-lens solution?" I wondered as we went to hide the bear bait.

Exhausted from our ten-mile hike, I collapsed in my sub-zero sleeping bag. Soon, John startled me, "Are you snorting?" he demanded in a low tone.

"What?" I replied, incredulously.

"I heard you snorting." I wasn't sure what snorting was until I heard it myself. The sound seemed about fifteen feet from our tent and it was intensifying.

"Snortt, snnuuggggfffm, thwummmppp." These weren't coming from me. We both knew what this was. This was a bear.

John whispered, "Don't move and don't talk, I want to see this bear." Why did we bother with the bear-proof canister if we were willing to be a main course? If we had our food at least we could give the bear a granola bar and run. This bear meant a lot to John. I tried to stay calm, but those reflexes kicked in. Flight or fight? This was not a test.

My flight response took over. "AAAAHHHHH," I screamed like a sissy girl. John couldn't reach the tent zipper through my flailing arms.

"Thwummmpppp, thwummmmmmp," was all we heard as the bear lumbered away. John was disappointed, but I couldn't help myself. A perceived threat to life outweighed his bragging rights.

Perceived. Would that bear have bothered us? The rangers told us black bears rarely attack people. But logic turns off in the midst of a dangerous situation. Were we in danger?

Our definitions of danger tell our bodies that doom is just around the corner. Running five minutes late for a parent-teacher conference is not going to kill us. But self-imposed stress will rob us of energy and make us sick.

Ginger Roasted Salmon with Asian Veggies

That bear should have been out looking for salmon, not our trail mix. This recipe actually reminds me of one of my favorite camp meals. A piece of fish roasted over a fire with vegetables. Easy on a campfire and even easier at home.

One medium salmon filet, about a pound

2 tsp fresh chopped ginger

2 tsp fresh minced garlic

2 TBS olive oil

2 TBS fresh lemon juice

2 TBS soy sauce

1/2 diced onion

1 cup sliced mushrooms

1 cup sliced red peppers

1 cup pea pods

Preheat the oven to 425. Lightly grease a baking sheet with olive oil or cooking spray. Lay the salmon filet on top of the tray. Combine the ginger, garlic, olive oil, lemon juice and soy sauce in a small bowl. Coat the top of the salmon with half of the mixture and let sit 10 minutes.

Ginger Roasted Salmon with Asian Veggies

(*Continued*)

Meanwhile, toss the remaining marinade over the vegetables and pour the vegetables onto the cooking tray, surrounding the salmon. Roast the salmon and vegetables 5-6 minutes then open oven and quickly stir the veggies. Roast another 5 - 6 minutes and remove from oven. Let salmon rest five minutes before cutting. Serves 4.

What Happened in That Tent?

Early humans needed to do one of two things in a life-threatening situation, take flight or fight. No one had to figure out if this month's numbers were going to put business in the red before being chased by the bear, they just ran for their lives or fought with their spears. Their decisions were based on physical survival, not mental state or a long to-do list.

When Pebbles Flintstone was running for her life, certain body functions kicked on to save her. The adrenaline rush I get racing home from Wal-Mart® so I won't miss the kids' bus was developed to save my life. Body responses turn on when we are threatened. But my life isn't threatened in the cat food aisle. And this is what is wrong with our stress response. It comes on too often.

Two major hormones are produced to save your life. Adrenaline is the one everyone knows. The people scaling the 3000-foot sides of the sheer granite walls of El Capitan in Yosemite Park thrive on that adrenaline rush. So do race car drivers and downhill skiers. Adrenaline helps them perform. This hormone is produced by the adrenal glands and it mobilizes sugar for energy and functions as a natural stimulant.

The other hormone that is produced when we're stressed is cortisol. This hormone also mobilizes sugar for energy (this is stored sugar) and it keeps us awake and alert. One of the big differences between these two major stress hormones is the length of time they stay active. You have probably felt adrenaline subside as you count to ten when your kids dump the container of flour on the kitchen floor when they decide to attempt making cookies by themselves. Adrenaline is the hormone that allows a parent to lift the car off his child, and unfortunately these superhuman properties quickly fade when the stressful situation subsides. But cortisol sticks around. Kind of like a watch guard. Your body just wants to make sure it's alert in case the bear circles back around. Cortisol levels can stay elevated for several days after the stressful event. You just never know what's around the corner. A beach vacation may be the only cure to lowering some people's constantly elevated cortisol levels.

When these hormones kick in, heart rate increases, blood thickens, perspiration flows, and muscle strength intensifies. All these responses are vital if you're going to run or fight. Non-vital functions like digestion and sexual responses stop so the body can send more energy toward self-preservation.

My body started to prepare when the threat of danger was perceived at the campsite. Increased heartbeat, check. Adrenaline flowing, check. Rapid breathing, check. Sexual function, it wasn't happening in the tent anyway.

All of the physiological responses that happen when you are stressed are meant to save your life. But they may end up killing you.

Stress Messes with Digestion

There is no bigger non-vital function than digestion. You can stay alive for 30 days without food and only about a minute without a beating heart. Digesting my **Butternut Squash Tostado** isn't going to keep me alive when the bear is after me. So my body adjusts. It stops making all the digestive enzymes that I need to break down food. And the food just sits...and sits. Think about it. If you remember, I said that about 50% of your energy every day goes to the function of digestion. Energy that you now need to outrun the bear. Only, now your bear is the deadline sitting on your desk. It isn't going to kill you, but it is going to give you a whopping case of indigestion. And indigestion is just the beginning of the problems.

With slowed digestion, important nutrients don't get broken down as usable fuel for cells to make energy. And while food isn't being used, it is causing problems. Think of all those chemicals that you ate when you opened that can of tomato soup and made a salad doused in bottled ranch dressing. Those food additives are sitting in your digestive tract, longer and longer as your body waits for the effects of stress to lessen. The number of cases of cancer of the digestive system, stomach, intestines and colon have risen rapidly in the past fifty years. Those chemicals that you ingest are being absorbed into your body as they sit for 36 to 72 hours longer than they should. And those chemicals have been linked to cancer and disease.

Digestion allows food to be used for energy. If you are not properly digesting because you are stressed, you don't get the benefit of the food you eat. And if you aren't digesting your food, you can have a host of other uncomfortable gastrointestinal issues. Ultimately, stress can lead to disease of the intestinal tract. And no one lying in a hospital bed is fully energetic.

Stress is Not Sexy

I was in a tent after hiking ten miles. Chances were good that we wouldn't be bumping boots that night. Even though it would have been a good form of entertainment in a quiet tent, it probably wouldn't have happened. Sex is a non-vital function. And after the bear incident my non-vital functions were on pause.

We only need to turn on the television or open any web page to know that a good number of the male population of this country needs a blue pill. And I hang out with enough stressed-out women to know that heading home to a long evening of love making isn't high on many of their lists. Our stress-filled lives have taken the spark away from many a relationship.

The hormones that need to turn on to produce the desire to have sex just don't get the signal. Sex hormones are produced in a number of places in the body. And one of these places happens to be the adrenal glands. Do you see something there? Adrenal? Looks like?

Yes, you got it, adrenaline. Adrenaline is produced in the adrenal glands. If those glands are overwhelmed with the production of stress hormones, then they are not adequately available to fill the purchase order for a few sex hormones. No delivery on that truck for you today.

If you want to revitalize a slump in your sex life, you need to take a serious look at stress in your life.

Stress Keeps Fat Sitting Still

The spare tire, love handles, muffin top. We all know what that refers to. The fat around the middle. This type of fat, for many, is the direct result of stress. Cortisol, that stress hormone that sticks around, has the capacity to deplete lean muscle and hold fat in place right

Butternut Squash Tostados
with Cilantro Yogurt Sauce

Cilantro Yogurt Sauce:

1/2 cup cilantro leaves

1/2 cup parsley leaves

3 scallions, chopped in ½ inch pieces, using half of the green part

1/2 fresh jalapeno, chopped (use the whole thing if you like spicy)

1 cup non-fat plain Greek yogurt

Juice of one medium lemon

1 tsp. cumin

1/2 tsp. garlic powder

Sea salt to taste

In the bowl of a food processor put the cilantro, parsley, scallions and jalapeno. Pulse for 1-2 minutes. Stop the processor and scrape down the sides. Pulse until fine. Add the remaining ingredients and process for 1-2 minutes until the sauce is well blended. It should be a lovely green color!

Butternut Squash Mixture:

2 TBS olive oil

4 cups chopped butternut squash – ½ inch cubes or less

1 medium onion chopped

1 tsp garlic powder

1/2 tsp onion powder

Salt and pepper

Butternut Squash Tostados
(*Continued*)

Preheat oven to 400. Pour olive oil on a baking sheet with sides. Toss the rest of the ingredients on the baking sheet. Roast the squash for 10 minutes and then stir with a metal spatula. Roast for another 10 minutes and stir. Continue this until squash is soft and beginning to brown on the edges. It shouldn't take any longer than 30 minutes. Remove from oven. Leave oven at 400.

Assemble Tostados:
Butternut squash mixture
1 avocado sliced thin
1/2 red pepper sliced thin
1/2 cup pepper jack cheese
1 recipe Cilantro Yogurt Sauce

Spray a baking sheet with non-stick baking spray (look for an olive oil based spray). Put 4-6 small corn tortillas on the tray in put in the heated oven for 3 minutes. Remove the tray and flip the tortillas over. Bake for another 3 minutes.

Remove from the oven and top each tostada with a couple spoonfuls of butternut squash, a few slices of avocado and red pepper and finally a sprinkle of pepper jack cheese. Put the tostados back in the oven and bake until cheese melts, 3-4 minutes. Top the tostados with cilantro sauce. Makes 6 tostados.

Kathy Parry

around the middle. It does this by increasing blood sugar during the stressful event. But when the exam is over or deadline is met, you will still have a high level of blood sugar. This excess glucose is stored as fat. And you say, "Hello, next hole in the belt!" I cringe when I see someone, especially men, wearing the same belt they did for the last twenty years. The worn marks at each hole show the gradual progression of belly fat. Time to stop stressing, reduce sugar and get a new belt!

Besides relocating fat to the mid-section, cortisol increases your appetite. Remember, if you're stressed from the bear your body is preparing you for a long run or intense fight. Therefore you're going to get signals telling you to eat. And because carbs convert most easily to energy, you're cravings will be for sugar. I call this the "How did I just eat a whole row of brownies?" effect. You don't even know how or why you did it. Your brain was signaling a need for carbs and you obliged your cranial urgings. I coach people all the time, especially women, who don't understand why they always feel hungry and unsatisfied. Increased cortisol levels are one reason.

In order to lose belly fat, and feel more energetic, you must take a serious look at your stress levels.

Stress is the Anti-Healer

I was talking to a friend who is a nurse at a local college health center. As a mother of college students I was curious about the peak time for illness. While visiting her campus I stopped in for a chat. It was mid-September and the campus was really active. I couldn't help but think about the adjustment that kids go through as they return back to school.

"So have you been busy?" I asked my friend over lunch.

"A little, but it's coming. It is definitely coming," she replied with a slight roll of her eyes.

"What's coming?" I asked, curious about what sounded like an impending storm.

"The six week mark. It always seems that it is just enough time for the stress, poor eating and no sleep to set in. It causes a huge wave of activity in the health center. We see it all the time. And then again right after finals. I think half the campus goes home sick for winter break!"

I wasn't surprised with her response. I thought about my own daughter who ended up with mono her first year of college. When she arrived home I promptly nursed her back to health with **Spinach and White Bean Soup**, lots of rest, and no reasons to stress. We usually know that lack of sleep and poor eating will catch up with us, but we are often unaware that those only pay a part in making us sick. Stress will make you sick faster than a week of burgers, fries and milkshakes.

Immune function is non-vital. At least in the short term. White blood cells don't get called up for duty when there is a bear to chase off. White blood cells operate on a couple different levels to keep out antigens, the bad guys. The bad guys come in the form of bacteria, viruses and cancerous cells. So living with some stress, like the kind that comes from finals week, can result in a cold or strep throat. But think if you lived with chronic stress. Your body's ability to fight off life-threatening cancer cells becomes diminished! Stress can kill you. And you have very little energy when you're dead.

Stress and the Big League Energy Zapper

My friend is a tough girl. Not just a normal tough girl, a tough girl who has a black belt. A tough girl who knows how to shoot a gun. A

Spinach and White Bean Soup

1 medium onion diced

2 cloves garlic, minced

2 TBS olive oil

2 carrots sliced

2 stalks of celery, chopped or sliced

1 medium zucchini, diced

3 cups chopped spinach

4 cups vegetable or chicken broth

1 15 oz can diced tomatoes

1 15 oz can white cannellini or navy beans

2 tsp dried Italian seasoning

1/2 tsp salt

1/2 tsp pepper

In a medium pot, heat the olive oil over medium heat. Add the onion and garlic and sauté until translucent, 5-6 minutes. Add all other ingredients and simmer 1 – 1-1/2 hours. Serve with my daughter's favorite sandwich, grilled cheddar and granny smith apples. (Put thin slices of apples right in the sandwich!)

tough girl who raised kids who don't misbehave, ever. A tough girl who works in Washington, DC with a lot of other tough people who think 60-hour weeks are the light shift. Tough.

Imagine my surprise when on a rare occasion she actually had time to call me.

"Hey, I can't believe you have time to talk!" I said excitedly as I was usually the one leaving a message.

"Oh I have all the time I need today," she responded, as I heard her exhale.

"What's going on? You don't sound right. Are you okay?" My own motherly instincts were kicking in.

"I don't know. I collapsed when I walked in from work a couple weeks ago, and I couldn't get up. Like literally couldn't get up all weekend. When Monday came and I still wasn't better I went to the doctor. He ordered a ton of tests. Nothing came up, no real illness I mean. But I was like dead, no energy. Finally he called and said he thought I was just burned out. Used the term adrenal fatigue. I think I'm finally coming out of it."

Wow, my friend took stress to the extreme. But then again, she was the only woman I knew to run a marathon just a year after giving birth! Adrenal fatigue is big league stress, not the wimpy scream-a-bit-and-eat-some-chocolate variety.

Adrenal fatigue occurs when adrenal gland function becomes less than optimal. Your adrenal glands cannot adequately meet the demands of stress. Whether you have an emotional crisis such as the death of a loved one, a physical crisis such as major surgery, or any type of severe repeated or constant stress in your life, your adrenals have to respond to the stress by producing the stress hormones. An estimated 80% of people experience adrenal fatigue and the physical symptoms of stress at some point in their lives, yet it is frequently overlooked and misunderstood by the medical community.

You may be experiencing adrenal fatigue if you regularly notice one or more of these symptoms:

- You're tired...really tired, for no reason.

- You have trouble getting up in the morning, even when you go to bed at a reasonable hour.

- You are feeling rundown or overwhelmed.

- You have difficulty bouncing back from stress or illness.

- You feel more awake, alert and energetic after 6PM than you do all day.

When you can't bounce back from stress and you suspect you may have burnt out your adrenal glands, the only real way to heal is rest. My friend, from the comfort of her sofa, was healing her adrenals. She definitely didn't have any energy to live an engaged and vital life. If you want to keep energy levels high, stress must be low.

How Can You Tame the Bear?

Stress leads us to make some unhealthy lifestyle choices. Why do you think Ben and Jerry's exists? In Chapter 7 we'll discuss emotional eating, but in order to tame the stress that is making us sick, we need to look at the choices we make when we are being chased. So besides that pint of Chunky Monkey calling your name, what can you do?

Acknowledge Stress

I love the weeks leading up to the holidays. Inevitably I will have at least one friend go off on how much they can't stand seeing certain relatives. I feel their blood pressure rising before me before the cranberry sauce is even set out on the buffet. You know that stress is coming. But how about the unforeseen traffic jam that is going to make you a half hour late for a meeting? That is a stress you didn't anticipate. So really there are only two types of stress. The one you know is coming and the one that takes you by surprise. In order to tame the bear, it is important to acknowledge and understand what you're going to do in either situation.

Let's go back to the Thanksgiving table. You know the preparation of the meal, the burnt Brussels sprouts, and your annoying uncle are all going to put you on edge. You know this. Don't sugar coat it a week before and say, "I'm not stressed at all about having thirty people for dinner." Instead, prepare. Have a plan for this event. We make all kinds of elaborate plans for major events. A wedding comes to mind.

My friend Kathleen was preparing for her daughter's wedding. I heard about the event for months. The details astounded me. It seems 25 years ago we didn't create a theme for the entire event, including the bird nest name holders with imitation eggs that read, "Love is so tweet." Really, Pinterest has created a whole new form of stress. But one lovely detail was left out in the planning of this wedding. A plan for stress. My friend was so exhausted and stressed out on the day of the wedding she admitted she didn't enjoy it as much as she thought she would.

When you know a stressful event or situation is looming, take time to make a detailed plan for your health. *Make a stress anticipation plan.*

Consider these questions the next time you're planning an event or will be a part of a stressful one.

- What situations may arise around this event that will cause me more stress?

- Do I have a plan on how to deal with those situations?

- Who would I call to help me? And who would respond immediately?

- What people at this event will cause me to feel stressed?

- What can I do ahead of time to ensure all items on the to-do list get done?

- What will I do after the event is over to ensure my stress levels are low?

After you've answered these questions, consider ways that you might keep stress low. If you have a situation that arises, who can fix it? At my own wedding the caterers didn't bring enough plates. The reception was at my home, and we wouldn't be there for several hours before the reception took place, so we assigned a family friend to arrive before the rest of the party to check on the caterers. Because we had thought ahead about situations that may cause us stress, we were all able to eat food off a plate. Yes, they had the logo of a local country club on them, but hey, they were quickly brought to the reception and without charge!

Holidays are big stress-filled events. And often it is the people at these events that get us wound up. Hey, you know every single year your uncle asks you why you don't have children yet. Or your brother harps on and on about his successful business and the European vacation he's taking his family on. Well, then have a plan. Be it avoidance, the world's best comeback line, or just some deep breathing; take precautions to avoid the stress of people.

The Great Unknown

The second kind of stress that you must acknowledge is that of

Not-Burnt Brussels Sprout Holiday Salad

My mother always burnt Brussels sprouts. We have no idea why. But of any food that would ever burn, it always seemed to be Brussels sprouts steaming on the stove. For her 75th birthday party, which fell just days before Christmas, I created this lovely holiday Brussels sprout salad. It looks festive, is filled with nutrients and doesn't have much chance to burn.

Peeling and steaming the leaves takes time, but alternatively, you can shred the Brussels sprouts whole by placing them in a food processor with a slicing blade.

1 pound of Brussels sprouts – individual leaves divided or shredded

1/2 cup pomegranate seeds

1/4 cup dried cranberries

1 green onion including some of the green – sliced very thin

1/2 cup slivered toasted almonds

the unknown. I know you're saying, "How do I acknowledge a stress that I know nothing about?" It is easy. Know that it will come. Stressful situations happen. We recently experienced some record rainfall and flooding. The people driving down the road had no idea that the road would soon disappear under a wave of water. Likewise, my neighbor walking down her basement, which had never had water in it before,

Not-Burnt Brussels Sprout Holiday Salad

(*Continued*)

Honey Vinaigrette:

1/2 cup extra virgin olive oil

2 TBS red wine vinegar

2 TBS balsamic vinegar

1/2 tsp Dijon mustard

1 TBS honey or agave nectar

Pinch of salt

Either individually peel each Brussels sprout into leaves or conversely, shred them in a food processor using a slicing blade. Add the Brussels sprout leaves to a vegetable steamer and steam for 2 minutes until bright green. Immediately run leaves under cold water. Add Brussels sprout leaves to a large bowl and add pomegranate, cranberries, onion and almonds. Put all dressing ingredients in a glass jar with a lid and shake vigorously. Toss just before serving. Serves 4-6

was unprepared for the stress of several inches. We may not know when stressful events will happen, but they will. So you must plan.

Often we look at these unforeseen stresses as a problem. Problems are difficult. Problems are bad. But if we rethink problems they become something of a different nature. One of my favorites quotes is: "You don't have a problem to solve; you have a decision to make."

Problems aren't fun. Decisions are. Think about how much fun you had trying to decide which pair of sandals you wanted to buy last summer. That's fun. So start thinking about the decisions you'll make the next time an unforeseen stress crashes your day.

Similar to knowing what stresses may arrive, ask yourself the questions below. Sometimes it helps to anticipate the situation that may arrive. For instance, if you know your parents are aging, answer these questions in the context of a phone call from a neighbor telling you that your mother was found fallen down on her driveway. Or if you have children, answer these questions as if they came home from school with a story of being bullied on the playground.

- When stress hits me unexpectedly, what is my first response?

- Do I call other people to help or do I handle it all myself?

- Who could help me in a stressful situation?

- Am I staying stressed for days over the situation or am I making critical decisions that will help the situation pass?

- Do I trust that all stress is under my control?

That last question is an important one. All our daily stresses are ultimately ours to control. After you have acknowledged the stress, the second step in moving through stress is to have a plan.

Get a New Plan, Stan

If you have truthfully acknowledged stress in your life, you should have a pretty good idea of how you feel when confronted with a stressful situation. The questions above should have prompted you to see how you deal with stress. Now, let's find out if you're dealing well!

If your first response to stress is something that involves yelling, drinking, or maxing out credit cards, then you may want to rethink your plan. All of these things may help you feel less stress, but ultimately are not the most healthful tactics.

Remember stress is affecting your health and energy levels. So it is best to get the situation under control quickly. One of the fastest ways to let your body know that the bear is gone is to simply breathe. It sounds too easy. But remember, your body needs to get more oxygen to the blood stream so you can run from the bear. Your breathing intensifies when the stressful situation presents itself. Your heart pounds, pumping blood to the extremities that need to help you escape. But you have the ability to override the systems that flip on during a stress-filled event. Just stop what you're doing. Stop the rushing, the yelling, and the frantic pace. Stop whatever your response may be and breathe. Take ten really, really deep breaths.

My deep breath day happened several years ago. I had my four kids in the car. I had to get two of them to activities with simultaneous start times. The third one looked pale and was complaining of a sore throat. I felt my heart race a bit and the adrenaline beginning to flow as the start time of practice came and passed on the car clock. "We're late! I'm going to be in trouble!" My daughter cried out as I pulled into her gym. This was competitive cheerleading practice for goodness sake, not the Olympic time trials! As I wheeled my Yukon XL into the parking lot I heard the beginnings of what I dreaded nearly every day. It always began with a bit of a yelp. Merritt, my youngest, was starting to go into a seizure in her car seat. Paige hopped out of the car as I unbuckled my seat belt. "Mom, what about my practice?!" JP yelled, as it appeared I was fleeing the scene. I opened the back car door and said, "JP, I think Merritt is about to have a seizure." Racing heart, fast breaths, adrenaline. It was all happening as I grabbed Merritt out of her seat and held her tight, hoping to calm the storm that was passing through her little body. This was nearly a daily occurrence, but always stressful, nonetheless.

As her convulsing eased, I placed her back in her seat. Knowing that the other children needed attention, I climbed back in the driver's seat. I was a little shaky. At that moment I told myself to stop and just be still a minute. I took one really long deep breath. That felt good. I took another. It wasn't until I had taken about six cleansing breaths that I felt calm. The storm was passing and I felt I'd gained control over the situation. My heart wasn't pounding. I had tricked my stress into submission.

When I took those breaths I was essentially telling my body that the situation had passed. Stop producing all those stress hormones and get on with life. Taking deep breaths should be the very first step you take in order to restore your body to a normal functioning mode. When you stop stressing, you allow your body to use energy in a productive manner, not draining yourself of energy used to fight off false bears.

Other methods for dealing with stress abound. Exercise is always at the top of the list because when you exercise you produce another set of hormones that often overrides the stress hormones. Some of the feel good hormones course through your body after a walk or yoga session. But mega-trainers beware. Excessive exercise can put stress on your body. During excessive training or even short bursts of high intensity workouts the body actually produces high levels of cortisol. Marathon runners often have high cortisol levels, which can lead to the host of problems discussed earlier. So the best exercises to eliminate the negative effects of stress and restore your energy levels are a walk, a swim, a low impact movement. These aren't the only exercises for good health, but they are good for de-stressing.

Food and Stress

Often the first thing we turn to when we're stressed is comfort food. Mine happens to be chocolate. Well, chocolate covered sea-salted almonds, to be specific. We'll discuss emotional eating at length in Chapter 8. But when thinking about stress, think about what you tend to eat when the bear starts chasing you. If it isn't something that falls into the healthful category, make a new plan. If you know you need crunchy foods when you're stressed, (which is very typical) then make sure to have raw vegetables available instead of chips. Pay attention to what you are putting in your mouth when you feel stress rising and make a new plan for the next time.

A Final Bear Story

On the same two-month trip when the bear came into our camp in Yosemite, we had an equally stressful bear situation in Glacier National Park. The bears in Yosemite are generally black bears. They usually don't eat people, just trail mix. But in Glacier, further north in Montana, grizzly bears roam the backcountry. As we were about to embark down a trail into the backcountry, loaded down with backpacks and a permit allowing us to be on the trail, we were halted at the trailhead.

"You can't go down the trail," a ranger said as he checked the permits that dangled from our packs.

"Our permit should be okay, we got them last night from the ranger station," I said with a questioning look.

"Nothing wrong with your permit," he responded, "But there was a grizzly bear attack up the trail about a half hour ago. A helicopter is due in to life flight the victim out. You'll have to go back to the ranger station if you want to hike in the backcountry today."

I watched as a team of rangers on horseback started down the trail. I felt my stress reaction kick in. It was amazing how just the threat of a bear could create the same response as an actual bear. That is what worry does to us.

The rest of the day, on a different trail in a different part of the park, I still felt the threat of the bear. I had a hard time enjoying the breathtaking views of jagged peaks and the smells of an alpine meadow. I was worried about a possible threat to my life. Worry is stress's best friend. In order to beat all aspects of energy-draining stress, you must not only avoid stressful situations, and know how to react when confronted by them, but you must also not allow the thought of the unknown to overwhelm your day.

The bear never appeared on that hike. I spent a lot of time worrying, as well as singing show tunes for a seven-mile hike. (Bears don't like to be surprised. If they know you're coming they'll usually get out of your way.) But I also missed a lot of the experience. Don't let the bears of life rule your day. Breathe deep, eat well, and stay energized.

Chapter 6

E

N

E

R

Get Sleep

Y

Crashing

I was sitting at my desk and I felt it. But I didn't acknowledge it. If your head is about to hit the desk, you don't really acknowledge it. You either catch yourself or your head goes down. My eyes were heavy and I was going down fast.

Remember the story of my junior high teacher at the beginning of the book? He hit the desk. My major head drop happened when I was about 28 and rising every morning by 5:15 to be at a job on the other side of the city by 7:00 am. About four o'clock one afternoon I was sitting at my desk back at home and my head hit the wood. I was out. Done. No energy.

I got on the phone later that night with my sister. Slightly refreshed from my brief nap, I asked her how she did it. She was a mother of three young children and she complained how she was always sleep deprived. "You just power through and nap when you can," she told me. I wasn't used to sleep deprivation.

Looking out my window from my bedroom as a teen, I remember languishing in bed. I would peer out the window, look at what the day seemed to hold, and roll back over. I loved sleep. In college I continued to sleep well and was the queen of the power nap. But my work schedule now was killing me. I felt drained and uncreative during the day. I had to figure out sleep or I was worried I'd fall asleep at my desk at work, or worse - maybe behind the wheel!

As a nation we are chronically sleep deprived. Who hasn't said or thought, "If only I had more hours in my day?" And unfortunately the way we find those hours is to rob them from our sleep bank. But like the best-planned heist, someone usually gets caught. And when we rob from our sleep hours, we end up the loser in a jail cell with disease, weight gain, poor immune function and let's not forget, a cranky attitude.

Star Trek and a Lesson in Sleep

Back in a nerdy part of my life I got a bit addicted to *Star Trek: The Next Generation*. I know. But The Food Network didn't exist yet so cut me a break. In a particular series of episodes a giant, evil entity known only as the Borg captured other life forms and used them to power its evil ways. So floating across the universe was this evil structure, fueled by life forms including humans who lost all of their own brain function and instead became part of the evil Borg, known as the collective.

Attempting to save their captain, who after a series of battles has been captured, the members of the Star Trek Enterprise entered the Borg and returned Captain Picard to the ship. Unfortunately, he was still brain numb. He has been assimilated into the collective conscious of the Borg and couldn't be questioned on how to disarm and destroy the floating cube that is the Borg. (Pretty nerdy stuff but hang in there.) But through a few spiffy sci-fi techniques, his crew is able to release just a bit of his brain from the clutches of the Borg. A blank-faced, ashen Captain Picard is able to mutter one word, "sleep." Assuming he is tired, the crew wonders if he wants to sleep. But one astute crewmember realizes that the captain is trying to send a message about how to disarm the Borg, and ultimately save Earth. "Sleep," Picard continued to mutter, as the crew calculated how to send a message, through Picard's brain, to the Borg to put the Borg to sleep. The command to sleep activated its regenerative cycle and powered down the Borg, allowing destruction of the space villain and saving humanity!

The Borg episode won an Emmy. Just saying.

We are not evil entities floating through the universe, but the story teaches an important lesson on sleep. The Borg places great value on sleep as being the only time when it can regenerate. During all other moments of existence, the Borg is using power to fight. We use our energy all day long to fight the good fight, love our families, work for a living, battle traffic, mow lawns, work out, solve problems...you get the picture. We use our energy all day long to live big lives. But if we don't go into a regeneration mode, we cannot win any battles (hopefully all for good!)

A Few Good Reasons to Sleep

It seems pretty basic. We sleep because we get tired. Believe it or not, scientists actually have come up with several reasons why we sleep. But I'm only going to share a couple of these theories because they have to do with energy. And that's what we're trying to find, right? The ultimate recipe for an energetic life! I feel almost silly saying this, but one of the secrets to having more energy is to get enough sleep. Something your mother told you for years!

Watching Nerdy Sci-Fi Chocolate Fruit and Seed Snack Bars

My kids love these bars. Yes they have some butter. Yes they have some sugar. But they also have lots of fiber, dried fruit and seeds. A lot healthier than a Twinkie for dessert!

Crust:
1/2 cup butter
4 oz apple sauce
1/2 cup brown sugar
1 cup rolled oats
2 cups whole wheat pastry flour
1/2 cup ground flax seed
1/2 tsp cinnamon

Topping:
1 cup chopped almonds
1 cup chocolate chips
1 cup raisins
1/2 cup chopped dried apricots
1/2 cup sunflower seeds
1/4 cup sesame seeds
3 eggs

Preheat oven to 350. Grease a 9 x 13 pan. Combine all ingredients for crust in a bowl; mix well. Press the crust into the prepared pan. Place all the ingredients for the topping in a bowl. Stir to mix well. Pour the thick mixture over the crust and spread evenly. Place pan in the oven and bake 18-20 minutes. Allow bars to cool on a wire rack before cutting into squares.

In Pittsburgh where I live, we have a few tunnels that lead into downtown. Periodically these tunnels need a repair. Do you really think the city would consider closing down the tunnel in the middle of the day for maintenance? Of course not. The big flashing signs appear around 10:00 pm announcing the overnight closure to fix ceiling tiles. You need to shut down your tunnel to get the repairs done that keep your cells and organs operating effectively.

So what kinds of repairs actually happen when you sleep? Well obviously when you're lying in bed with the flu, you sleep. Your immune function needs you to rest so it can get to work. In other words, some of your systems are powered down so the immune system can get its work done. But besides being ill, other important functions are repaired and restored only during rest. Muscle growth and tissue repair happen during sleep. Protein is synthesized when you sleep and growth hormone is only released at night. Could you imagine a pre-teen trying to hit a growth spurt if they never slept? And now it becomes clear why babies sleep, they're doing a lot of growing!

So Energy Conservation and Restoration are two of the biggest reasons we sleep. But what happens when that sense of peace and shut-eye elude us? We are tired, body functions are impaired, and we set ourselves up for disease. Yes, sleep is that powerful.

What Happens When We Don't Sleep

This isn't the 1700's and most of us don't live on the tundra. We have electricity. Artificial light, as well as cable TV, have led us to mess with the Energy Conservation Theory. We fight our natural instinct to sleep at night and instead we power up with all available means electricity. We watch television into the wee hours, we work night shifts, and we pull all-nighters studying for biology exams. Fighting against this natural instinct to sleep leads to sleep deprivation.

95

Sitting in the basement of my dorm sophomore year I was faced head on with a decision. Stay up to study Accounting 101 or face the consequences of being unprepared for my exam. I chose to pull the all-nighter. And who hasn't? As the hours ticked by I tried all the tricks: caffeine, stretching, candy, and short bursts of frantic exercises. At about four am, I dropped my ten-pound accounting book on my finger. I started to cry. I was melting down amidst my debts and credits. My head hit the desk and I felt helpless. Heading to the exam on an hour of sleep didn't prove to be my best tactic. Accounting and I were not friends ever again after that. I focused on my Food Management classes instead and never pulled another all-nighter.

When we're sleep deprived even for a short period of time a cascade of physiological effects happen. In studies where subjects are only allowed four hours of sleep for four days, the impairments to their health and wellbeing began after only one sleep-deprived night. One of the first things to go is memory. This does not come as a shock to me after my Accounting debacle. In the studies, subjects were exposed to a new task in the afternoon and then had a good night's sleep. These people were able to remember the task with a higher degree of efficiency than those subjects who had four hours or less of sleep. So poor memory is one of the first markers of sleep deprivation. But that is only the beginning of a downhill spiral brought on by lack of sleep!

Did I Really Eat That?

When sleep deprivation becomes normal for even a short number of days, you get hungry. Yes, the munchies set in. You may wander out of bed and meet up with Little Debbie® in the kitchen. Or maybe it's a bowl of cereal every night at 3:00 am. I have a friend who says she never even remembers what she ate when she eats in the middle of the night! This need to feed is a direct result of too little sleep.

When we're sleep deprived our levels of a hormone called leptin are reduced. If you don't know leptin, let me introduce you. This spiffy little hormone is the hunger hormone. It has a few different functions. It stays on the lookout, surveying your energy balance, and then turns on your munchies or tells you to keep your hand out of the cookie jar. But when you aren't getting enough sleep, leptin levels drop. Signals are sent that you need more energy and your body knows that if you're not getting sleep, a midnight meet up with Ben and Jerry's might do the trick. Funny how those middle of the night snacks are never kale and carrots.

Midnight Munchies Kale Dip

1 cup plain Greek yogurt

2 TBS mayonnaise

2 cups kale, chopped fine

1/2 cup chopped red pepper

2 scallions chopped

1/2 tsp onion powder

1 tsp dried dill

1/2 tsp garlic powder

1/2 tsp salt

Combine all ingredients and serve with vegetables.

Maybe you aren't a midnight snacker, but you still see the number on the scale rising with no real explanation. Sleep deprivation can lead quickly to weight gain. Let's have a review of Chapter 5 – the look at stress. Your body views sleep deprivation as stress. And guess what gets produced in higher levels when we don't sleep? Cortisol. And if you remember from Chapter 5, cortisol is one of the hormones that tell our body to hold onto fat. This is a self-preservation method gone awry in our sleep-deprived world.

So in two different ways chronic sleep deprivation can lead to obesity, which in turn leads to a whole host of chronic degenerative diseases.

A Cascade of Crazy

Besides poor memory and weight gain, the domino effect of chronically sleeping less than seven hours a night can produce mayhem in daily life. I have first-hand experience down a slippery slope to crazy. And it came wrapped in a tiny bundle. Babies equal sleep deprivation.

Baby number three, Graham, was the toughest on my sleep patterns. After number one, Paige, and number two, JP, arrived, there was always an opportunity to nap, because everyone napped. When my two-year old and baby napped, Mom napped. But by the time my third child arrived, Paige was four and JP was two and we rarely had naptime. No, bouncing off the walls, grabbing toys from each other, and drawing on the table with markers was more their style. After about a month of night-time feedings that resulted in four to six hours of sleep per night, I started to get loopy.

I was never one to yell at my kids but I found that the slightest thing set me off. And I wasn't just being set off emotionally; I was literally *off.*

Waking up at 1:00 am and then 4:00 am and then getting up for good at 7:00 am, I stumbled a bit and grabbed JP's hand as we walked slowly down the stairs. He was 2-1/2 and demanded Cheerios® and a cup of juice filled to the filled to the "tippy" top as soon as his feet hit the kitchen floor. The baby was still asleep for the moment and Paige was playing in her room. No doubt the budding fashionista was scattering five mismatched outfits across her bedroom floor. I filled JP's juice, and went to set it on the table and promptly knocked it over. I couldn't even blame him, it was all me. I felt like such a klutz as I cleaned up the mess and watched JP splash in the mini juice puddles on floor. Just as I was wringing out the dishtowel filled with juice, Paige came down the stairs.

Paige immediately began to taunt JP. It was harmless stuff, really. She was trying to mother him and his host of stuffed animals into a makeshift pre-school. "Bossy" is the word that comes to mind. But when Paige grabbed JP's favorite stuffed Little Bear from his arms, I knew we were in for problems. Little Bear stayed firmly attached to JP until about noon each day. Screams erupted. As the tug of war proceeded I felt my stress level rise. I asked them to stop. I walked over, threatening time out. The warring factions had no interest in mediation. The toddler war escalated. Paige pushed JP to the ground. His head conked on the hardwood floor just as I reached the front lines. I didn't think. I just reached out and smacked Paige's face. What?

I had never hit one of my children. It wasn't a parenting tactic that I had ever planned to use. Both children turned their eyes to me and Paige began to bawl. What was I turning into? I put both children in time out chairs and promptly removed myself to my own time out corner. Time to think this one through.

Sleep deprivation and all of its ugly symptoms had taken up refuge in my battle-weary body. I was clumsy and emotionally volatile. Everything set me off. Simple tasks felt labored and making dinner seemed as difficult as cooking for a five star restaurant. I knew if I didn't get some sleep soon, the cascade of crazy was going to turn my rather calm demeanor into a woman who terrorized neighborhood children and dogs. Everyone had quiet time that afternoon and I slept without guilt.

So Just Go to Sleep

If sleep is so critical to our energy levels and health, then why don't we just do it? As I said before, we try to add hours to our days by robbing from the sleep bank. That is reason number one. Until you decide that sleep is more important than *Dancing with the Stars* or finishing your expense report, you'll probably never feel fully rested. Sleep must become a priority if you want to stay energized.

But maybe your schedule isn't the issue. Maybe you've tried to go to sleep and you just can't. A vast number of us toss and turn and pace all night. What's up with that? Why do we pop so many sleeping pills in this country? One of the simplest answers to that question is: the bear. Remember my story of the bear in the last chapter? When the bear is constantly after us, our stress hormones will not allow us to sleep. So reducing stress is one of the first things you can do to get more sleep.

But stress isn't the only thing keeping us up. Diet is a key factor in how well we sleep. Different foods and the way we digest are both reasons for sleepless nights. A few years ago my father was complaining of restless nights. It wasn't until he cut his afternoon iced tea habit that he began to sleep better. The caffeine late in the day had never affected him before, but suddenly it was the culprit. And I had a friend who had gotten into an after dinner ice cream habit. She didn't realize the two or three bites of coffee ice cream she'd been sneaking after dinner had enough caffeine to keep her up. And I've had my own midnight

Five Star Crock Pot Lentil Sloppy Joes

Kids, buns, sloppy…what's not to like? If you have never embraced the ease, nutrition and value of lentils, here is a perfect place to start:

1 cup dried brown or green lentils
1-1/2 cups vegetable broth
1 15-ounce can diced tomatoes
1/4 cup tomato paste
1 onion, chopped fine
1/2 red or green bell pepper, chopped fine
1 TBS apple cider vinegar
2 cloves fresh minced garlic
1-1/2 teaspoons oregano
1-1/2 teaspoons smoked paprika (don't skip this)
1 TBS chili powder
1 tsp sea salt
Freshly ground black pepper

Stir all ingredients together right in the slow cooker. There's no need for measuring cups, just eyeball or get out the kitchen scale for the lentils, broth and tomato paste! Cover and cook on high for 3 - 4 hours or on low for 7 - 8 hours. Check for consistency, it might be necessary to take the lid off for the last 30 minutes or so.

Serve in buns or as a side dish. Keeps for a week or more, and is easy to rewarm.

madness when I've eaten chocolate after dinner. Certain foods with caffeine or sugar can cause some sleep disturbance.

But besides just the foods we eat, the manner in which we eat them can cause us to stay awake or worse, wake up at 3 am, never to sleep again! In Chapter 3 I discussed the role that sugar plays in digestion. Adding sugar at the end of any meal can lead to digestive problems that keep you up at night. And many people who are up in the middle of the night try to calm their gurgling stomachs with - yes, you know...more food! We think we can calm a stomach with more food. What really may help at this point is a high quality digestive enzyme supplement. These natural enzymes help break down food and speed digestion.

Other reasons you may not be able to sleep range from cold feet (yes, a study actually showed that if your feet were cold it was several times more likely that you wouldn't sleep well) to a full moon. But one of my favorite studies about sleep, or rather lack of sleep, deals with the weekend. My friend used to call it a weekend hangover. And she wasn't talking about tailgating with a keg in the back of a truck. When her children were young, their family schedule was so chaotic on the weekends that their normal bedtime routines were a mess. Pushing the kids to stay up so they wouldn't have to leave a family party, getting them up early the next morning for soccer games, and eating junk along the way all led to a big, old cranky disaster on Monday. It generally took her whole family several days to restore their sleep habits to a normal pattern. And then it was time for another weekend. You don't have to have young children to experience disturbed sleep patterns. Anyone who travels for business, is trying to meet deadlines, or becomes enthralled with the latest Robert Ludlum thriller can interrupt their body's normal rhythm. Keeping a sense of routine with sleep habits is a key to getting a good night sleep.

Twinkle, Twinkle Little Star

Leaning over their sweet-smelling, post-bath foreheads, I used to linger at my children's bedsides singing three lullabies. It was always three. They had me suckered into three because I just loved the smell of those clean kids. Lullaby number one was always silly. I made up a song about the trash truck and sang it every night to my boys. Bedtime song number two slowed down a bit, usually Barney's theme song or a Sunday School song, but song number three...that's when the magic happened. When *Twinkle, Twinkle Little Star* began I could see their entire bodies relax. Their eyelids got heavy, yawns were common and I knew I had the golden ticket, sleepy kids.

A sense of routine is a great way to ensure easing into a good night's rest. It works just as well for adults as children. Going to bed at roughly the same hour is the start of the routine. But after that, each of our routines is different. I knew one friend who fell asleep with her iPod under her pillow every night. She couldn't have in earbuds, she had to hear the music through the pillow. Another friend had to set a glass of water next to her bed and read for exactly fifteen minutes. Sleep habits can be as ceremonious as pre-game rituals before your team's biggest game. Honor those habits and keep them constant if they help you fall off into a good night's slumber.

Tossing and Turning

A few years ago a very popular song by Uncle Kracker called *Smile* captured my attention. In the first stanza the line, "You're cooler than the flip side of my pillow," actually made sense to me, and probably most of us. When we're trying to fall asleep we'll try anything. And flipping over the pillow to get a cool sensation seems to be a very popular tactic. The song is cute, but tossing and turning at 2:00 am is not.

So what do you do if sleep eludes you? If you've tried to de-stress and you still aren't able to sleep, I'd like to offer a few suggestions that may help. Sleep is a funny thing and so much of it is based on our production of key hormones. Hormones are the messengers of the body and one of their jobs is to signal the body to sleep. But if you are not producing the right hormones, due to stress or a variety of other reasons, you will have difficulty sleeping.

One of the first steps I encourage people to try is visualization. Think of a place. The most peaceful place you can conjure up. My place is under a pine tree in the middle of the woods. I have a huge down comforter, I mean like twelve inches thick. When I'm lying in bed, unable to sleep, I go to this place. If I really get into my visualization, I can smell the forest. No one else is allowed in. I'm only allowed to be still in this place. No bears trounce through my spot. No thoughts are permitted to fill my mind; just the feeling of what is surrounding me. Then I breathe. Just like when I am stressed. I take ten deep breaths. This visualizing and breathing work wonders to relax me.

The power of visualization is impressive. In fact I bet after reading that last paragraph you may have even felt yourself relax. Pick your place and give it a try. You may be surprised that even without a cross-country trek or expensive airfare to the islands you still have the ability to be someplace relaxing.

If you're still tossing after twenty minutes try what I call the heavy-hand technique. While still visualizing your spot and lying down, raise your hand up in the air. Keep it there for a minute or two, until it literally starts to feel heavy. Your arm is tired. You are tired. Then slowly, like inch-worm slow, lower your arm. This lowering technique may take a minute or two. By the time your arm hits the bed you should feel a great sense of relaxation flow through your body. Go back to visualizing sleeping in your quiet spot.

Still tossing? Well on nights when I know I'm stressed and feel that sleep may not be my friend, I use a supplement called melatonin. Many people use melatonin to help encourage sleep or regulate jet-lag. Melatonin is not a sleeping pill but rather the hormone that your body naturally produces to tell you it's time to sleep. But again, when you're stressed or not making hormones efficiently, you're not going to produce melatonin. So sometimes we can trick ourselves with a synthetic version of the stuff. For me it works. And whenever I take it I have some really vivid dreams, which is kind of a bonus because I love to wake up remembering a crazy, good dream.

Happy Nappy

When I was about thirteen I began to indulge in the habit that many teens, babies and octogenarians live by; the nap. Naps are a way to get caught up on some sleep, but studies show that we must have that long-deep restful night sleep to stay healthy. But I still live by the nap. I try to get my 7-8 hours of sleep, but like most people, sometimes that just doesn't work. But boy a twenty-minute power nap on the sofa is sure a sweet way to refresh. I had a friend in college who was a pro at the library nap. I'd walk by his study spot and see him out cold in a chair. Sometimes our bodies overrule our busy schedule and just tell us to sleep. And that is usually a sign that we aren't getting enough sleep at night.

I encourage you to take a serious look at your sleep patterns. If you are not consistently getting full nights of sleep, consider making sleep a priority. Skills and memory are affected by lack of sleep and over time vital organs become hindered when the body does not have time to restore and repair.

At about the same time I discovered the power of a nap, I also realized how nice it felt to sleep in on the weekends. Forget my childish ways of waking at 6:00 am on Saturday to get a jump on the Saturday morning cartoons, nope! My teen years were meant for staying up late and sleeping in later. While staying over at a friend's house I made the statement, "Let's sleep in really late," as we turned off the lights around 2:00 am. My friend's reply still sticks with me today, "I hate sleeping in; I don't want to miss my whole day." And that is unfortunately what drives a lot of our sleep behaviors. We don't want to miss out on life. But until we realize and honor the vital role sleep plays in our health and energy levels, we may set ourselves up to miss parts of life we never imagined. Now go to bed!

Chapter 7

E

N

E

R

G

Your Plan

The Best Laid Plans

My friend Julia was pregnant. And she was a planner. A pregnant woman with a plan can make remarkable things happen. It takes nine months to grow a baby and most women need that long just to plan for the arrival. Nesting instincts kick in and nurseries are painted, baby sleepers are washed and breastfeeding classes attended. And Julia was no different. The nursery was painted lavender, pink blankets neatly folded, and the name Alexandria was picked. But then Alex arrived. And Alex would be wearing blue. We don't always get to choose the plan.

I'm a planner. Okay, I'm an over-planner. I like a good checklist. A reminder set in my phone. An itinerary. Plans get things done. But sometimes our plans get foiled. In no other realm of life is this more apparent than our health. We may start off with the best intentions, to eat real, whole foods all day long. We start the morning with a fruit and kale smoothie, pack a lunch of chickpea salad. But about two o'clock someone says, "Cookie tray in the break room!" And we are suddenly reduced to a no-plan wonder. Or how about that plan to get to bed earlier? Get the sleep you know your body needs. But then you find a Seinfeld episode you forgot all about and you're hooked into not one show of Kramer scheming to open a smoking lounge in his apartment, but also a second episode when Jerry forgets his date's name. Soon it's midnight and you know your head will be drooping at your desk tomorrow.

I'm going to guess that over 90% of everyone reading this book knows what they're supposed to do to feel well and energized. Well actually *everyone* reading because I've just covered it all! Lots of vegetables and whole, real foods, limit sugar, avoid junk, reduce stress and get sleep. But somewhere along the way all that information gets muddled and the greatest sabotage of our health takes over. Emotions. Yep. Our emotional turmoil or even emotional exuberance has turned us into a nation of chronically tired and overweight individuals. In order to live a vital and engaged life, you're going to have to figure out your relationship with food, stress and sleep. I've given you a few pointers on planning for stress and sleep in previous chapters. But now I'm talking about a food plan. A plan with defenses against emotions. But, before you can plan, you have to understand your obstacles.

The Obstacle in the Road

When I drive down a major thoroughfare near my home I stare at the eyesore that was Hollywood Video. Yep, an ugly façade that looks like a torn movie ticket sits empty. Slowly decaying, the yellow and red sign speaks to an era that came and passed rather quickly. Video stores like Blockbuster® and Hollywood Video® used to be staples in every town. When my children were preschoolers we'd go to Blockbuster and rent *Barney's Big Adventure* brought to us on a VCR. By the middle school years all the VCRs were gone and we headed out to rent *Harry Potter* on DVD. The stores were keeping up with technology, overcoming obstacles. But all that was before live streaming, DVRs, Hulu® and iPads®. When these stores opened, who could have imagined a day when we wouldn't drive to rent a movie? Sitting in front of your laptop and having Jack floating through the Atlantic on the *Titanic* as he declared "I'm the king of the world!" was unimaginable.

The onslaught of digital technology was an obstacle to the movie rental industry. And most didn't adapt. Netflix® and Redbox® seem to be the sources that did adjust, but that's probably because they didn't have expensive real estate tying up their assets. They simply had to change their distribution formula. But the depreciating asset that was the former Hollywood video store serves as a reminder: overcome your obstacles, or become an aging, decrepit relic. Now when I drive by the vacant store I just think, "Why can't Whole Foods go in there?"

So do you know and understand your obstacles to your diet? Are new shiny foods your issue? Do you clamor for the latest food trend? For the majority of us, knowledge about what and how to eat is not our major hurdle. No. Rather, the mistake of eating the disaster called the Doritos Locos Taco from Taco Bell is wrapped in a package of complex emotions. Yep. ***Emotional eating is the number one reason we are an overweight, un-energized nation.*** It's time to slap a smile on and learn why your emotions may be getting the better of you.

I'll Second That Emotion

Seventy-Five percent of all eating in this country is emotional. Think about it. Could you cut 75% of what you eat? No, not really. But what you're choosing to eat is based on emotion about 75% of the time. When you head out to lunch after a busy morning, do you think that mac n' cheese at the diner down the street would sure taste good right then? We think about the taste of food and how it will make us feel. And the majority of us aren't thinking about **Quinoa Salad with Tomatoes and Zucchini** as comfort food, but maybe we should.

Quinoa Salad with Tomatoes and Zucchini

Quinoa is a nutty grain from South America that cooks quickly and is full of nutrients and protein. Use it as a base for these classic summer combinations.

1 cup quinoa, cooked according to package and cooled (This should yield 2+ cups cooked)

1 cup chopped fresh basil

1 clove garlic chopped

2 cups diced tomatoes or cherry tomatoes

1 cup shredded zucchini

1 cup fennel bulb, chopped fine

1/2 cup olive oil

Juice of one lemon

1/2 cup feta (optional)

1/2 tsp sea salt (or to taste)

Pepper to taste

Cook the quinoa according to the package and cool. Add the basil, garlic, tomatoes, zucchini and fennel to the quinoa. Toss until well combined. Drizzle the olive oil over the salad and add lemon juice. Toss well. Add feta and salt and pepper to taste. Serves 4-6

Our emotional food decisions are based off of two sets of responses. One is called Head Emotions. These are the feelings that come after you get stuck in traffic, trying to get your mother to a doctor's appointment, after you've taken the morning off work, and then you wait for an additional hour in the waiting room for the next available time slot. When you finally leave the appointment a couple hours later, only to hit rush hour, you get home and open a bag of chips. Ahh.

When emotions like stress, anger, and frustration enter our day we often look for foods that crunch or are chewy. This chewing action allows us to relieve some stress. Foods like chips, M&M's, pizza, cookies and popcorn all allow us to chew away some of that pent up head full of emotions.

The second set of emotions that are an obstacle to healthful eating are the Heart Emotions. You may feel these emotions the day that your daughter forgot your birthday and no one is available to celebrate...not even your dog! You're feeling lonely, unfulfilled, depressed or bored. These are the days when ice cream may become dinner. Other comfort foods we go for are cheese, cinnamon rolls, donuts, pasta, and chocolate desserts of all varieties!

When I begin to work with coaching clients often they ask if I want them to keep a food journal. I already know that they aren't eating well. They wouldn't be sitting across from me if they ate creamed kale when they were lonely. Instead of a food journal, I suggest thinking about an emotional eating journal. Every time a food goes in your mouth, ask yourself "why?" Assign this bite an emotion. What are you feeling right in that moment and what other activity could you do to help you through the feeling?

You actually don't have to start a spiral-bound, leather-covered journal of food and emotion, but keeping a running list of emotions for about a one-week period is very revealing. Make a list of the following emotions: anger, stress, frustration, loneliness, sadness, feeling unfulfilled. You can come up with some of your own, too. Run the date down the side of the page. When you've found that you just pounded three handfuls of peanut butter-filled pretzel nuggets, stop. Think about if you were actually hungry and if that was the best option? Or did an emotion drive you to stick your hand in the bag? After about a week of conscious eating, you should see some patterns emerge. I crunch almonds as soon as my stress level goes up. You might think, "well, that's pretty healthy." But if I'm crunching handful after handful of almonds without being hungry, they aren't serving much more purpose than adding calories, which can add weight and zap energy as I work all morning to digest.

After you've identified the emotions that lead you to eat, begin to plan some alternate activities that could fill that emotion gap. Feeling lonely and unfulfilled seems to drive the late night ice cream habit for a lot of people. Yours may be something other than ice cream, but evenings spent alone or without a sense of involvement may be easy to treat with a phone call to a long-time friend or even a little connecting on Facebook. Join a club that doesn't have a sole purpose of eating. Sometimes we just so badly need other people in our lives and without that connection, food becomes our friend. If the head emotions are more your trigger point, try a walk around the block or some meditation when you feel the stress or anger rising. Sign up for an evening exercise class. Food will never be the companion you need to fulfill an emotion. It will end up stabbing you in the back, heart, liver and gallbladder, just to name a few.

Snackalicious

If 75% of our eating is emotional, then the majority of that eating doesn't happen when we sit down to a meal, with a napkin, with real silverware. No, we snack. We have become a nation of snackers. From the 1970's until present day, we've added the equivalent of one full meal of calories from snacks. Last Christmas Eve I was sitting in church. Three young children sat with their parents in front of me. Every one of the children got out a bag full of crackers and fruit gummy snacks during the service. No time is sacred. We have a need to feed. Cars, planes, bathrooms, waiting rooms. When I'm in public and look around, I see people eating. Gone are three meals a day. We eat all day long.

So we've talked about the emotional side of eating, but how do we curb our desire to snack? Some additional tactics to have in your plan concern the way you snack.

First, know when you get hungry. Assessing your need to eat should be one of the first steps to making your plan. If you work out at 6:00 am are you always starving by ten? Are the drive-thru and an Egg McMuffin® calling your name? Or do you know that as soon as you walk in the door from work you always need to eat? Start taking note of what hunger feels like. We're allowed to be hungry. And when you are hungry, a lot more foods taste good. I've climbed several 14,000-foot mountains in Colorado. When I get to the top after four hours going straight up at high altitude, I'm starving. A handful of trail mix tastes like an amazing treat. Begin to plan your snack times based on hunger, not emotion. Keep track of the times you feel the hungriest and be prepared with a meal or snack.

The second part of that preparation is to pick the appropriate snack. Ask yourself, "Is my snack nutrient-dense?" A carrot is better than a cupcake. We know that. So implement that thought when snacking. I was coaching an older gentleman on his diet. He said, "You aren't going to make me give up my two-a-day rum and Coke® habit are you?" First of all, I don't ask anyone to do anything. If you want to make changes, that is all on you. I may hold you accountable to the goals you set, but I can't pry the Bacardi® out of your hand. So I asked if he could begin to move towards a drink that is more nutrient dense. Say, a rum and orange juice, and then maybe give up that habit and move toward a glass of red wine. You don't have to move from snacking on Cheetos® to only eating cucumber slices. Maybe you like peanut butter and crackers. Try almond butter on an apple or pear instead. Look for the foods with nutrients! You'll soon see that incremental changes will make a difference on the scale and in your energy level.

And a final tactic when making your snack plan is to understand how much you need. Portions are out of control in this country. Walking past the glass display cases at any chain bakery/café reveals quite a bit about our eating habits. When I was a child a muffin was about two inches across. At these bakeries the muffins are about four inches wide. And that is one of the reasons we see so many muffin tops on women and beer bellies on men.

But there is also a reverse-psychology marketing plan happening on our grocery shelves. It comes wrapped with the labels, "mini" or "bite-sized." Yes, we've completely bought into this marketing scheme. If we take a Snickers® bar and reduce it first to "Fun Size" and then even further to "Bite Sized," well then surely we've taken a bite out of all that is bad with big candy bars! But who eats just one? Okay, you may eat one at a time, but it has been proven that if these mini treats are left out in a bowl, most people will eventually eat the equivalent of a full sized candy bar over the course of a day. And it isn't just candy bars that are being marketed as mini. The 100-calorie packs of a wide variety of snack foods have us thinking that these are a great alternative. Heck, a banana has 100 calories, but we go for the mini Oreos instead. This is yet another time when your "nutrient dense" reminder should go off! The 100 calories in the mini bags are full of a mini amount of nutrients! Eat the banana.

Another tactic for portioning is getting a bowl. Bowls are essential because they keep your hand from continuously dipping into a bag or box. And don't use a soup bowl. Go to your local cooking, housewares, or even Asian food store. All of these places will have a wide variety of small bowls. I bought some at an Asian market that are the perfect size to hold a few ounces of nuts or a half a sliced apple with some almond butter, or a couple cubes of cheese. The big bowl is out for food portioning.

Another step to portioning involves looking at the label. I'm not a huge fan of a manufacturer defining how much you eat, but at least you can see the calorie, fat and sugar amounts in a suggested serving. But again, just because the manufacturer recommends an amount, that doesn't mean you need to eat that amount. Certainly don't go over it. I think it is wonderful how nature portions. A whole fruit or vegetable is a nice portion. Well, maybe not a whole head of cauliflower, but apple, orange, banana, carrot, red pepper, even a stalk of broccoli are all portioned to eat whole.

Winner Winner, Chicken Dinner

Fine. You get snacking, emotional eating and portions. But, what happens when it's time to sit down to a meal? Somehow we've come to understand that three meals a day need to grace our tables. And this stresses a whole lot of us out. We don't like to cook. We don't like to shop. We don't like to chop up vegetables. The local chain restaurant thrives on our decision to skip the meal preparation. Skip the grocery store on Thursdays...there's always TGI Fridays®!

Sorry, but the only way most busy people can make a whole foods lifestyle work is to have a plan. In a recent lecture I actually had a woman roll her eyes at me when I mentioned meal planning. The contempt I feel from some people when I ask them to plan is amazing!

But if you arrive home from work at 6:00 without a plan, you, like any other hungry species, are going to go for the path of least resistance. You're going to eat what's easy. The lioness on the savannah goes for the gazelle that is 50 yards away, not the one 200 yards in the distance. Meal planning allows you to bring whole, real foods closer to your plate.

The number one excuse I get for not making dinner is: **I don't have time!**

Really? Because I think at the max you should consider a good, healthful meal to be about an hour commitment. And if you're smart, you can cut that time in half. Think about all the different events in your day to which you commit an hour. How many of them serve your health? How many of them are detrimental to your health? How many of them are important to you? Is an hour watching *NCIS* helping you feel energetic?

If your best friend had to have an outpatient procedure and really needed a ride to the hospital and someone to sit for an hour, would you do it? If your son's team needed an extra parent at a practice to hand out uniforms and make arrangements for the upcoming tournament, would you do it? If your daughter called from college in tears, aching from a breakup, would you stay on the phone for an hour to help her through it? And if your father needed some help putting the storm windows in this weekend, could you find time? We often find the time. A good friend gave me a valuable lesson on how to find the time you may be missing.

When I was pregnant with my second child I was sitting with a bunch of other moms in a church gym hoping to get an extra-long naptime by allowing our toddlers to run around like wild animals. Dinner was the hot topic in this circle of new moms. One friend looked at me and said, "You will never cook dinner once the second child arrives!" Wow, was it really that time consuming? Another friend, who knew I liked to cook and had a pretty healthy thing going on said, **"You will always make time for what is important to you."**

Is your health important to you?

My guess is that all those other people in your life who demand pieces of your time are not the only ones who are important. You are important. It is okay to take the time to plan for a whole foods lifestyle. Why do we think it's okay to make time to go to the doctor, sit in the waiting room, go for tests, and get prescriptions filled, but we have a problem with sitting down to make a plan for healthful eating? In order to live a vital and energetic life, you're going to need to plan.

Get a New Plan, Stan

When Julie Andrews wanted to teach the VonTrapp children how to sing in *The Sound of Music*, she said, "You must start at the very beginning." And if you want to teach yourself how to get real, whole foods on the table that starting place is making a plan.

When my children were young I had some planning issues. As in, they wrecked all my plans. Anyone with young children knows what I mean. When you have toddlers and babies and cats and husbands and schedules it is hard to plan meals. But it isn't just moms with young children; school, careers, volunteer activities and practices all take a chunk of our time. As a vegetarian, my own food preferences focused on fresh produce. The only way to get fresh produce is to grow it or buy it and the aforementioned distractions kept me from tending a garden. So I had to find time to buy some food. Seems basic. But with young children, the prospect of grocery shopping was about as fun to think about as having wisdom teeth pulled. I knew my lack of a plan was leading me down a bad path the evening I caved and served chicken nuggets and tater tots. Really, was this the best I could do?

117

I got out a notebook. That's what planners do. Well, you can also use Evernote® or Google Keep® or a wide variety of virtual planning tools. But I like a notebook. After a pathetic stretch of busy nights and uninspired family meals, I knew I had better face the music and plan some meals.

I made two columns in my notebook. On one side of the page I put, "Grocery List." On the second half of the page I put: M, T, W, Th, F, S, S. A whole lot of empty stared back from that page. Then I just began to think. What did my family like to eat? What were my time constraints? When could I shop? Wow, this was a whole lot of questions just to get food on the table. But soon I was filling in the blanks. And a beautiful thing emerged. A plan. I knew that we usually ate chicken once a week and pasta once a week. Whew! That was already two days taken care of. Next to Monday I put chicken and next to Tuesday I put pasta. I continued to think about my week and to picture what would work. Thursdays seemed like a good day for fish. Fridays became "Fun Food" day. This was the day I reserved for foods like tacos, (with kale in the meat!) pizza, (with whole wheat crust!) or Parmesan-coated chicken nuggets (recipe in Chapter 4!). Soon every day had a food either assigned or a category designated. For a while my family was really into Mexican food, so Wednesdays became Mexican-inspired. Quesadillas, enchiladas, even a layered Mexican casserole became favorites. And the beauty of all those foods is that vegetables like shredded zucchini are easily hidden within! So my first most difficult step to meal planning was solved. I had a formula that simply needed pieces plugged in. I could probably come up with 10,000 chicken recipes pretty easily with the help of the Food Network. I would never worry about what to eat on a Monday again!

I've used this model for years. And it wasn't until about three years into the schedule that someone actually noticed that we had pasta on Tuesdays. I mixed the variety up enough that meals did not repeat with much frequency. And soon my kids, who were now all school aged and a bit food savvy, began to make requests for certain days. My favorite day of the week became Sundays. In the summer the food assignment for Sundays was burgers. Now these took many varieties: hamburgers, salmon burgers, black bean burgers, crab cakes. But then once the air turned cool, Sundays became soup day. I kept a running list of about twenty soups taped inside one of the cupboards. After Sunday dinner was over, one child would be chosen to open the cupboard door, peruse the list and choose next week's soup. And the kids became more aware of soup recipes and asked me to try new ones. My plan for next Sunday was done!

You may not be dealing with a young family. Maybe you have a house full of teens who never know until a half hour before they're starving if they'll even be home for dinner. Or maybe it is just you and a spouse and some unforgiving schedules. You may feel that you have huge obstacles in your way when it comes to meal planning. But if you sit for just an hour and really think about your lifestyle, time constraints and favorite foods, a plan will begin to emerge.

Please go to my website: www.KathyParry.com for your planning tools. Here you will find worksheets that will guide you through a meal planning session. You'll be asked to think about your family's likes and dislikes. Come on, your doctor asks for a complete family medical history when you show up, doing a food history for your family isn't a huge task. And the goal here is to keep you away from the doctor, keep you energized and enjoying your vital life. **Take the time to make the plan.**

The grocery store was the next obstacle to the plan. I realized I had to make a plan just to get to the store. Because visiting the mega-market with three children led to a cart full of bribes and missing ingredients, I knew I needed time alone. Some people long for a few quiet hours to read, I just needed to find an hour or two undisturbed to shop. I was rescued by pre-school. Oh what a lovely concept. Once a week the stars aligned and my older two were in preschool and Graham, my number three, was just old enough to go to a church-sponsored mother's morning out program. But this doesn't just happen to moms with children. I coach a number of young professionals who never seem to find the time to grocery shop. Making an appointment to shop is the key. We all have snazzy little smart phones with apps and functions and bells and whistles. Program in your shopping like it's an important appointment. Armed with a list, a plan for meals and the time to do it, I set off to shop.

The Next Food Network Star

I like to cook. I like to cook a lot. So the cooking part of the food wasn't a big deal to me. Finding the time was a bit challenging, but I can throw together **Indian Spiced Chick Pea and Lentil Stew** in ten minutes and be done. But I know that cooking isn't everyone's gift. You may not be the Next Food Network Star, but there are so many tools available to make cooking easy. In the grocery store you can buy the vegetables already chopped. Already chopped, did you hear that? And the internet is full of recipe sources and meal planning sites. The issue again becomes the plan.

One fall when my children were in 8th grade, 6th grade, 3rd grade and of course Merritt who was at home, my well laid plans took a hit. The three older children were all involved in numerous activities that seemed to fall during the dinner hour. On Tuesdays I was basically in the car from 3:30 to 6:30. One Tuesday evening while getting ready to take Graham to his practice and pick Paige up at her gym, it dawned on me that Graham hadn't eaten since his after school snack of an apple and some pretzels. I had a dinner planned to make around 6:00 but realized Graham wouldn't be back until 7:00! He needed something to

Indian Spiced Chick Pea and Lentil Stew

This is a great dish to put on the stove a couple hours before you plan to eat. Bring it to a boil then turn it on low. Additional vegetables of your choosing can be added to the stew, and a couple cut up chicken breasts can be added too.

2 TBS olive oil

1 medium onion chopped

2 carrots chopped

1 cup chopped kale

1 15 oz can tomato sauce

3 cups chicken or vegetable broth

1 15 oz can organic chick peas

1 cup green lentils

1 tsp cardamom

1 tsp cumin

1 tsp curry powder

1 tsp garlic powder

1/2 tsp salt

Black pepper or red pepper flakes to taste.

Heat olive oil in a large deep-sided skillet over medium heat. Add the onion and sauté for 3-4 minutes. Add all the other ingredients. Simmer over low for 1-1/2 - 2 hours. If stew becomes too thick, add more broth or water. Adjust seasoning before serving. I like my food spicier so I add red pepper. Serve with a dollop of Raita Sauce. Serves 4-6.

Indian Spiced Chick Pea and Lentil Stew

(*Continued*)

Raita Sauce

1 cup non-fat plain yogurt (Greek or regular)

2 TBS chopped fresh mint, or 1 tsp. dried

1/4 tsp salt

1/4 tsp cumin

1/2 tsp honey

Combine all and serve with lentils.

eat and I'd forgotten him. (Truth be told, this was not the first time I'd forgotten Graham. Number three child also once got left at soccer practice...hard to keep them all straight!) However, from that day on I reworked my plan. Until the fall schedule let up, pasta day would be postponed. On Tuesdays, everyone got a wrap. Sometime earlier in the day I would make turkey or chicken wraps, fill them with shredded red peppers and carrots (always hiding those veggies) a bit of cheese and condiments. I would wrap them in foil, take a Sharpie marker and write each child's name on the outside (and usually draw a funny picture) then throw them in the fridge. Now they would have something to hold them, or even serve as dinner, that had some nutrients. Our days are always changing and we need to adapt.

One form of adapting is what I call Emergency Meals. I encourage you to always have the ingredients for three to four Emergency Meals on hand. These are meals that can be prepared in thirty minutes or less. This works well if you're fond of stocking up. I actually sometimes feel like a food hoarder! Several years ago we were buried under a record three-foot snowfall. We had no power for 36 hours. But I had a gas range a stocked pantry and freezer full of food. I managed to make dinner and lunch for my family and a couple neighbor families as well. Dining by candlelight was a fun way to spend the storm-filled days.

A snowstorm is one type of food emergency, but really any random Wednesday can turn into a mess. The **Stuffed Acorn Squash** that you had planned to serve could easily fall by the wayside when you get stuck in rush hour traffic that involves a jack-knifed semi-truck. You roll into your garage with a plan that no longer works. Of course pizza works. Right? That's the first instinct of many time-deprived people. But it isn't the most healthful option and certainly won't leave you feeling full of energy for the night. Nope, pizza at the last minute usually leads to some stress eating and a whole lot of energy loss. This is when the second type of Emergency Meal comes into play.

Several years ago I was returning from a weekend wedding. It was Sunday night, we were exhausted and I didn't have much energy to make a big dinner. Not to mention the kids were hungry and it was soup night. Instead of opening a can, I concocted **Spinach and Orzo Tomato Soup**. It was done within the thirty-minute parameter set for Emergency Meals and it was full of more nutrients than a MSG-filled canned option. Learning to keep on hand the ingredients you need for a few emergency meals is key. Wraps or pita pockets filled with shredded veggies, quick soups, stir-fries, omelets, etc. With all the frozen vegetable options and high-quality sauces, throwing something together is pretty easy...as long as you have a plan.

Stuffed Acorn Squash

This recipe takes a bit of baking time, but it is a perfect main course on a fall evening.

1 acorn squash split in down the middle, top to bottom

1/2 pound silken style tofu

1/2 tsp cinnamon

1/4 cup dried cranberries

1 TBS olive oil

1/2 cup walnuts or pecans chopped coarsely

Salt and pepper to taste

Preheat oven to 350. Fill a shallow baking dish half way up the sides with water. Place the split acorn squash cut side down in the water. Bake at 350 for 45 minutes or until soft when pressed on the skin. Scoop the squash out of the shell and put it into a medium sized bowl. Add the remaining ingredients and stir to combine well. Put the rice mixture back into the squash and reheat in oven for 10 minutes. Serves two as a main course or four as a side.

I adore Trader Joe's®. If you don't have a Trader Joe's market near you, I'm sorry. Really I am. You're missing out on a fun food experience. But stores like Trader Joe's along with rival food market, Whole Foods®, do an excellent job of stocking quick and easy meal ingredients that don't contain a lot of the chemicals found on many of the conventional grocery store shelves. An easy way to make an Emergency Meal is to use a quick sauce or condiment. But I urge you to stay away from national brands. Fake foods are everywhere. But if you're lucky enough to have a Trader Joe's nearby, try the Thai Yellow Curry Sauce with steamed vegetables and a piece of fish. That takes all of about fifteen minutes to prepare, especially if you get one of the many assorted chopped vegetables available in the produce section.

Some people lay out their clothes the night before. No surprise-ironing or outfit changes for these fashion planners. But when I turn out my light, and lie in bed for those few minutes before I doze off, I think about the events of the next day. And I make sure I know my food plan before I go to sleep.

Spinach and Orzo Tomato Soup

1 15 oz can tomato sauce

1 15 oz can diced tomatoes

1 cup water

1/2 package frozen chopped spinach, defrosted

1/3 cup dried orzo pasta

1 tsp dried Italian seasoning

1 tsp garlic powder

1 tsp agave nectar for sweetness (or a 1 tsp of sugar if you don't have agave)

Combine all ingredients in a medium-sized saucepan over medium heat. Bring to a simmer. Allow soup to cook until pasta is soft. Serve with a sprinkle of Parmesan and red pepper strips on the side! Serves 4.

But maybe part of the food plan is picking a place to eat. Hey, that's okay. Nobody said you had to don an apron and cook every night. But eating out means we give up some control over what we eat. It's time to make a plan for this too. Write down your favorite places to eat out. Is the list long on fast food? Fine dining? Mid-priced chains? Think about why you go. Do you really enjoy the food or are most of your restaurant meals just for convenience? After you've figured out why you eat out, think about what you eat when you go out. What are your go-to meals? Go ahead. Take a break and make a list of your favorite restaurants and what you like to eat there.

After you've assessed what and where you're eating, think about making it better. If it's a Mexican place, could you replace the beef enchiladas with their vegetarian version? Could a bowl of black bean soup and a salad work? And here's the big question...could you ask them not to deliver chips and salsa to the table?? (Or at least not ask for a second basket!)

Almost all chain restaurants now list food content and provide a degree of labeling for their menu items on their websites. If you're eating out, check the website before you leave. Make a plan before you enter the restaurant. Or how about this: pick a new place. Yeah, that's right. Try some Indian, Chinese, or Thai. These nationalities base their diets on plants. Since becoming Americanized, many of them use more meat, but you can find a lot of healthful vegetable options.

Get a bit outside your comfort zone. If you've always chosen a fast-food burger chain, try a place like Chipotle instead. The options at some of the newer chain restaurants are fresher and healthier. Burgers and pizza are our national standard for quick and easy meals out. And unfortunately our obesity levels reflect that.

Party Hardy

Snacks and dinners aren't the only eating events that are important to plan. Even though snacking on a bag of chips can be detrimental to your health, just stepping into a party is one of the biggest obstacles we face in our plan. No, I'm not taking away your right to party. I love a social outing as much as the next person. But for some reason, party food generally isn't healthy food. Opening your home, basement or venue to guests often means throwing health to the wind. When my friend Renee labeled cupcakes as "Party Foods," her young children understood they were reserved for those fun times. And most tailgates and graduation parties I've been to don't have a big bowl of **Chia Seed Crisps** next to **Red Pepper Salsa**. No, the big take-to-your-next-get-together-dish I keep seeing pop up is Buffalo Chicken Dip.

My dear friend brought this dish to a family gathering where ten teenagers were in attendance. Those teens descended on the dip as if they were fruit flies on a rotten banana! A concoction of canned chicken (ugh), bottled ranch dressing, cream cheese, blue cheese, and hot sauce make up this party delicacy. (But look on page 131 for my **Buffalo "Chick" Dip**...my teenage boys ate this like it was the junk version!) This apparently tasty treat is full of artificial chemicals, saturated and hydrogenated fats, and almost no nutrients your cells need to stay healthy and energized. Yet, it's a party! And just because of that...we go for it!

Unless you've been invited to your vegan friend's, Dr. Oz's or to my house, the party is an obstacle to your plan. Knowing and understanding the obstacle needs to be part of your plan. Begin to think of parties as social events to connect with people you're interested in and not as a place to stuff your face. Part of your plan may be to make a list of all the people you want to have conversations with. Talking leaves a lot less time for eating.

Chia Seed Crisps and Red Pepper Salsa

Yes, Chia seeds are the same ones used to grow hair on a clay Chia Pet®. But other than making a cute plant to sit in your window, Chia seeds are a true super food, loaded with nutrients. These crackers are fun to make and give a nutrient dense, gluten free alternative.

1/2 cup chia seeds

2 cups water

1/2 tsp. salt

1/2 cup pepitas (pumpkin seeds)

1/2 cup raw sunflower seeds

1 tsp. garlic powder

1 tsp. Italian herb seasoning

1/2 tsp red pepper flakes (optional if you don't like some heat)

Preheat oven to 350. In a medium sized bowl combine the chia seeds and water. Let this mixture sit for about an hour or until it turns into a thick consistency. Stir occasionally to minimize any chunks.

Meanwhile pulse the pepitas and sunflower seeds in a food processor until coarsely chopped. Add the chopped seeds to the chia mixture. Add the salt, garlic powder, herbs and red pepper. Spread parchment paper on a cookie sheet with sides. Spread the chia mixture thinly across the parchment. It is okay if some holes appear. Try to get the layer of chia mixture as thin as possible using the back of a spatula.

Chia Seed Crisps and Red Pepper Salsa
(*Continued*)

Bake at 350 for 30-45 minutes. The baking time all depends on how thin your chia mixture is spread. The crackers are done when the edges and top are browning and the entire thing feels crisp. Remove from oven. Allow to cool, then break into pieces. Serve with red pepper salsa.

Red Pepper Salsa

1 whole red pepper, chopped in 1 inch pieces

3 medium tomatoes (about 3 cups) chopped in 1 inch pieces

2 green onions, chopped in 1 inch pieces

1 TBS. red wine vinegar

1 tsp. cumin

1/2 tsp. salt

1 handful of cilantro leaves

1 avocado, cut into six pieces

Put the red pepper, tomatoes, and green onions in the bowl of a food processor. Pulse until quite fine. Add the vinegar, cumin, cilantro and salt and pulse to combine. Finally, add the avocado and pulse for 5-10 seconds until chopped but not pureed. Makes approximately 3 cups salsa.

A second part of the plan could be to eat before you go. Yes, it's okay not to eat the food at the party. I get a lot of flak for this. People are constantly trying to get me to eat. I know I can appear to be a food snob, and maybe I am. But it shouldn't be considered rude not to eat. You are making decisions for your health and energy levels. Your host or hostess or Great Aunt Mary shouldn't guilt you into a serving of Triple Chocolate Layer Cake. The best tactic I've found is to eat something I enjoy before I go to a party. Once arriving at the party, pick one or two things you know you'll enjoy and then eat a small portion of them. And most parties will at least have some vegetables cut up and sitting lonely next to the bratwursts and beer. Enjoy those.

Of course if the event is a sit down, four-course dinner or a wedding with table service, not a buffet, the planning dynamic changes. If I'm faced with this type of dinner, I often call the venue. I find out what the menu will be and ask if they can arrange for a special meal. Don't bug your host or hostess or even the event planner, just call the caterer, club or hotel direct. Ask to speak to the kitchen manager or chef. With the numerous food allergies and special diets people are adhering to, chefs get this all the time. Upwards of 10% of all people attending events now request a special diet. So find out what's on the menu.

I was once attending a women's conference with over 300 attendees. A simple phone call landed me with a lovely plate of hummus, mixed vegetables and whole wheat pita wedges for my lunch. A few people looked on enviously as they worked their way through a creamy looking chicken salad on a croissant. But if you want a special meal, don't wait until the day before! If it is a private individual hosting the event, like a wedding, make sure your host won't be charged extra. Your special requests shouldn't put a strain on your friendships...you may not get invited back!

Buffalo "Chick" Dip

1 15 oz can organic garbanzo beans

1/2 cup crumbled blue cheese

1 cup plain, non-fat Greek yogurt

1/4 cup buffalo hot sauce (I used Franks brand)

Put the garbanzo beans in the bowl of a food processor. Pulse until rough chopped. Add the blue cheese and pulse several more times, until fairly smooth. Add yogurt and hot sauce. Pulse to combine. Transfer to an oven-proof dish. Bake at 350 for 20-30 minutes. Serve with celery and pita chips. Makes 2 cups. The dip can also be served cold!

And speaking of friendships, this is one of the final obstacles in your plan. In the book, *The Blue Zones*, by Dan Buettner, the author talks about the habits of the people who live the longest. He studied areas of the world with the highest concentration of centenarians. That's 100 years and older, or a whole lot of great, great grandmas! One of the areas he studied was the small Italian island of Sardinia. It turns out on Sardinia the men in the villages gather every afternoon, often to enjoy a glass of red wine but also to laugh. The author points out many reasons why this island hosts an older population, including a plant-based diet accented only a bit with meat, important family values, walking almost five miles daily on average and that important time with friends. I've known several people who have failed miserably at making a plan for better eating just because of the people around them. If you want to succeed at gaining more energy and living a vital and engaged life, you should consider the people already in your life.

If your friends insist on wings, pizza and ice cream as a fun night out, it may be hard for you to get the support you need to make your plan. An honest conversation with the people who you care about most in your life is a good place to start. If your family doesn't support your need to make changes, this can also be an obstacle to making a plan.

Don't try to change everyone's attitudes overnight. Small subtle changes work best. Families are rough because they can be your toughest critics. I once left the table in tears after a boycott of bulgur wheat tacos. (I will admit, they weren't that great.) But I kept at it. When my daughter was seventeen and declared she wanted to try to be a vegetarian for a month, I felt a tiny bit self-satisfaction. And she did it.

Research from the Framingham Studies showed that smoking, obesity, happiness, and even loneliness are contagious. So the centenarian's health behaviors are favorably shaped by the people in their lives. We want to fit in. But it's important to find the right people to fit in with. If you don't have people in your life who may support the changes you want to make, do what we do whenever we need an answer. Google it. In most towns and cities there are Meetup® Groups. Just "Google" Meetups and your city. Put in healthful eating or vegetarian or weight loss. Local libraries, grocery stores and cooking schools often sponsor events about food and healthful eating. Invite me to inspire your group with a dynamic lecture! (Go to www.KathyParry.com to learn more about my speaking events.) Make it part of your plan to become in tune with where the healthy, energetic people hang out. If you're going to live an engaged and energetic life, you'll need to find some people to share it with!

Chapter 8

I'm Still Tired! Can't I Just Take a Pill?

But What If I'm Still Tired?

You've learned that in order to stay vital and energized you should:

Eat Energizing Foods – A Whole Foods, Plant-Based Diet

Not Sugar and Caffeine

Eliminate Fake Food

Reduce Stress

Get Sleep

Your Plan – Made and Implemented

Even though you may be well on your way to changing habits and implementing your plan, you may still be feeling tired. What's that about? I am not a medical expert so I can't tell you the exact reason you may still feel tired. The host of reasons for a body feeling fatigue ranges from an extra-long workout yesterday to a slow, but steady degenerative disease growing inside you! Yikes. Not to scare you, but if you have been feeling chronically tired, meaning weeks on end with your head dropping on your desk or nearly falling asleep at the wheel, you may want to visit your doctor for some blood work. It could be something as simple as nutrient deficiencies. But it could be something more serious. Let's talk a bit about the nutrients we're not getting.

One of the most common nutritional deficiencies that lead to a tired feeling is a deficiency in B complex vitamins. And B12 is the most common culprit. This vitamin produces energy from the metabolism of

133

fats and protein. Energy...it's an energy vitamin! But some of us don't get it. And I may be one of them!

B12 is one nutrient that is scarce in a vegetarian diet. And this becomes an interesting argument from all my meat-eating friends, but especially my seventeen-year-old son, JP. JP is on the debate team. He really likes meat, and dislikes the lack of meat in meals I serve. The kid can win an argument about almost anything. Debate team sounds like a group that would keep your kid out of trouble after school while they study how to argue the pros and cons of the rise of the Chinese economic system. I was thrilled with his choice of extracurricular activities. Until I realized I had to go up against his debating skills on everything from car-driving rights to my vegetarian lifestyle. "So if we were meant to be vegetarian, then why would you need to take B12 supplements?" he asked. Valid point. Here's what happens. B12 is actually produced by microorganisms in the intestinal tracts of animals. So the majority of people get their B12 from an animal source. However, plants can also take up B12 if grown in B12 rich soils. But our soils are barren and often over-farmed, so very limited amounts of B12 ever get absorbed by plants. So, JP, if we hadn't over-farmed our vegetables, and if vegetarians only ate vegetables grown in a garden that was fertilized with cow manure, then we wouldn't need to supplement with B12.

Some people who are low energy opt for B12 shots. The funniest thing happened while I was giving a lunch lecture on energy at an advertising firm. I was talking about the subject of B12 and someone from the back of the room shouted out, "You can get twelve B12 shots for $99.00 on Living Social®!" I laughed out loud. So now our lack of energy is being addressed on a discount social site. Most people are getting B12, but many aren't absorbing it.

B12 is a vitamin that can only be digested by your body through high stomach acid content. It takes a lot of acid to break down this essential vitamin. BUT, in this country we shut down our stomach acid production. Remember the information in Chapter 3 about digestion? Sugar and junk foods mess with digestion and we in turn take a whole lot of acid reducing medication. Acid in the stomach isn't the problem. We're supposed to produce stomach acid. It breaks down food. The problem is over-producing it to keep up with the crazy diet we're putting in! Eliminate the sugar, reduce the fried foods and get your digestive system back in order. Then, your body will break down the B12 and you'll feel energetic and not have to be poked in arm with a B12 shot!

At this point you may start thinking, "Hmm, if B12 makes energy and meat has B12 then I should increase meat in my diet for more energy!" Sounds like a good logical point. But you're dealing with a person who eats a plant-based diet and has more energy than most people half my age (and I've learned a few debate skills from my son). So you're going to get a bit of a shock when I tell you, we eat way too much meat in this country and we don't need it.

When my eighty-year-old father talks to me about how I'm feeling he loves to rib me by saying, "Why don't you eat a little meat? You would feel even better!" And that is a very normal American mentality. In this country upwards of 30% of our calories come from protein. And most of that is animal-based protein. But really, for health and vitality we need only 8-10% of our calories from protein. People constantly ask me, "Where do you get your protein?" A handful of almonds, some hummus and some beans are enough to meet my percentages. Also, a whole lot of foods besides a rib-eye steak have protein. Even vegetables and grains have proteins. But my original question was about B12. In my opinion, the benefits of eating a whole-food, plant-based diet far outweigh the negative effects of animal protein in the diet. So because our soils may not adequately supply plants with B12, I do supplement with this nutrient.

At this point I could launch into some very pointed and specific reasons to adopt a vegetarian lifestyle. That isn't the intent of this book. I have done the research for what works best for me and how I feel most energetic. Becoming a vegetarian is not the same as eating a whole-foods, plant-based diet. Some vegetarians eat cheese fries and drink orange soda. These vegetarians also lack a lot of energy because they are not getting the nutrients they need and their bodies spend a lot of energy digesting and detoxing that junk. So in all honesty, I'd rather have you decide to eat a clean diet, full of nutrient-dense foods and maybe an occasional grass-fed beef or **Blackened Wild Salmon Burger** than become a pizza and mac n' cheese-eating vegetarian!

All In That Little Gland?

So B12 deficiency, either from poor absorption or lack of the nutrient, could be an issue for fatigue. Another culprit in the quest for more energy is a quiet little butterfly of a gland known as the thyroid. This small gland nestled in your neck doesn't look like much, but if it isn't working right it is sort of like your furnace going out on a sub-zero day. Can you make it through your day? Sure, put on blankets, light a fire, eat some soup. You'll come up with a way to feel warm until a repair happens. But you won't be too comfortable.

The thyroid gland excretes hormones that can travel to every part of the body, including the brain, where they can affect mood, energy level, body temperature, metabolism, development and growth. If a thyroid becomes "sluggish," meaning it is underactive, it results in a condition called hypothyroidism. Some symptoms of an inefficient thyroid include: tiredness, weight gain, depression, and memory loss. You can live with symptoms like that, but like a broken furnace, you won't be too comfortable. Those are not markers of an energetic lifestyle!

Blackened Wild Salmon Burger

I do occasionally eat fish. And salmon is one of the most healthful fish, but make sure it is wild. Some farm-raised salmon actually has red food dye added. These fish are also not fed a natural diet.

1 – 1-1/2 lb. fresh or frozen wild salmon

2 eggs

1/2 cup good quality breadcrumbs

1 recipe blackened seasoning (recipe below)

2 TBS coconut oil

1/2 cup plain unflavored Greek yogurt

1 TBS organic mayonnaise

1 tsp organic ketchup

High quality whole wheat buns

Blackened Seasoning:

1 TBS paprika

1 tsp salt

1/2 tsp pepper

1/2 tsp cayenne pepper

1 tsp garlic powder

1 tsp onion powder

1/2 tsp dried oregano

1/2 tsp dried thyme

Combine all ingredients in a small flat bowl.

Blackened Wild Salmon Burger

(*Continued*)

For the salmon patties:

Fill a shallow sauté pan at least half way up the sides with water. Heat the water over medium high heat until it simmers. Do not bring to a boil. Add the salmon to the water and poach for about five to eight minutes. Set salmon aside to cool for ten to fifteen minutes until it is easy to handle. Crumble the salmon into a food processor and pulse two to three times. Add the eggs and breadcrumbs. Pulse until the salmon barely comes together. Form the salmon into two to four patties, depending on how mush salmon you used, and place them on a plate.

Heat the coconut oil over medium high heat in a sauté pan. Take each salmon cake and place it in the blackened seasoning. Turn burgers over to get seasoning on both sides. Put burgers into hot pan and sear. The seasoning will turn dark; try not to burn it. Cook on each side approximately 3-5 minutes.

While burgers are cooking, combine the Greek yogurt, mayonnaise and ketchup. Season it with the leftover blackened seasoning. Do this to taste, but generally 1 – 2 tsps.

Serve salmon burgers with a dollop of sauce, lettuce and tomato. Serves 2-4.

But how do you get a misbehaving thyroid? A poor diet can tax your thyroid. The thyroid needs several vitamins and minerals to keep functioning at an optimal level. Some of these include Vitamins A, D and E, selenium, iron, zinc, copper, omega-3 fatty acids, iodine and B vitamins. Remember my illustration about the emergency room and nutritional triage? The thyroid is just a gland sitting in the back of the emergency room with a cut needing a stitch. It isn't a heart pumping blood to the whole body or a liver in charge of detoxifying and aiding in digestion. In other words, our thyroids are non-vital; they aren't an emergency. Or are they? Fatigue, weight gain and depression don't sound like the best way to live a vital and engaged life, do they? But our bodies are only concerned with the trauma patients when there is a nutrient shortage. Our critical organs get the nutrients and our thyroid doesn't. Some foods that you may consider eating for thyroid health include nuts, seeds, sea vegetables and avocados. Avocados have a powerful antioxidant called glutathione that strengthens and repairs thyroid tissue.

So lack of nutrients is one reason your thyroid may be making you tired, but your thyroid may be losing steam for an even more insidious reason. This is the stuff that makes me crazy because most of us don't see it or understand it. Chemicals are affecting our energy levels. Scientific studies show that chemicals found in products we use every day may be damaging our thyroids. Perfluorooctanoic acid (PFOA) is an industrial chemical used to make nonstick cookware, microwave popcorn bags, stain-resistant clothing, and many other products. PFOA does not readily break down and is now found in the bodies of many Americans. Research has linked PFOA to low thyroid activity, and some animal studies have found an association between PFOA exposure and thyroid tumors in rodents and monkeys. Another chemical that has been linked to hypothyroidism is triclosan, which is found in everyday items like antibacterial soaps, toothpastes and fabrics.

139

If you think you may be suffering from an underactive thyroid, the best place to start is with some tests done by an endocrinologist. In the meantime, it is always best to limit your chemical exposure. We need to begin to question the chemicals we inhale, ingest and absorb. The chemical soup that we mix into our cells everyday has a wide and varying effect on our health and energy levels.

Can't I Just Take a Pill?

Some of this information is overwhelming. In lectures I've had people say, "It's just too hard. I have no idea what to eat. Can't I just take a pill?" I sure wish I were paid by the number of times I'm asked that question. We're lazy. We want the easy way to good health. Why is the supplement industry a 32 billion dollar industry? Because we want the easy answer to feeling well and being energetic. We want to pop a pill and not eat kale. We want to be youthful, energetic, skinny, wrinkle free, healthy, and with the sexual vigor of twenty-year-olds. Nutrition doesn't come in a pill. Aging is inevitable and doing it well takes more than a pill.

One of my favorite things to do is check out grocery carts. Okay, so if you see me at the store you will now run and hide your Fruit Loops® and Oreos®. But honestly, I think we all do it. We wonder, "Now, what is she going to do with that Marshmallow Fluff®, four bags of frozen peas, three boxes of Pop-Tarts®, and smoked sausage?" Peering into those rolling carts of crappy combinations makes for some interesting thoughts. And hey, I know I'm not off the hook. When people run into me at the store, the first thing they say is, "Don't look into my cart!" And then they immediately peek into mine. I know they're thinking, "Does the wellness chick really eat well? Let's just see if there are any chips." (Sometimes there are!) But my favorite place to look into carts is at the warehouse stores. Sam's Club® and Costco® are a statement on consumerism, temptation and mega-portions. The carts at the warehouse clubs are a good read on the state of our health. And by the number of mega-supplement jars going into the carts, many of us think these potions will make up for the plastic tub of pork rinds nestled next to the cheese curls.

Cruising into Sam's Club on a Saturday, I immediately hit the type of traffic that flows through the tunnels into downtown Pittsburgh at rush hour. I was bottlenecked at the barbeque. I don't make a habit out of going to Sam's Club on a Saturday, but I was nearby and needed avocados. I like some of the deals on produce at the mega center. (They sell an organic mix of baby kale, baby swiss chard and baby spinach that makes the most amazing **Mixed Sautéed Greens**!) So I'm halted by a group of shoppers stopped by the free samples of pre-packaged, pre-cooked pulled pork barbeque. And I'm sort of mesmerized. Free. Free causes a lot of poor decisions. Just because they give you a paper tasting cup filled with free food, doesn't mean you should load your cart with the chemical-filled entrees and snacks. But back to my trip. As I try to chart a course around the back up, I swing towards a giant display of supplements. Everything from ten-inch high jars of fish oil to a year's worth of Vitamin C, all piled into towers. Two women stand contemplating the fish oil. And I can't help but listen in. "You need this. This is what you take for your heart. And I think it prevents cancer too. Dr. Oz says we should take fish oil and he's a heart doctor." Her friend throws in a mega bottle.

"Hmm," I think as I peer into their carts. Family-sized strip steak tray, three-pound packages of ground beef, three blocks of cheese, two or three boxes of assorted crackers and cookies, frozen pizzas, chicken nuggets...the list could go on and on. The one place these two middle-aged, overweight women didn't seem to stop was the produce section. But jumbo fish oil, "check."

Mixed Sautéed Greens with Avocados and Red Peppers

1 red pepper, chopped

6 cups assorted, chopped greens (spinach, chard, kale)

1-2 TBS. organic coconut oil

1 avocado chopped

1/4 cup raw pumpkin seeds

1/4 cup raw sunflower seeds

Sea salt

Trader Joe's African Smoke Seasoning or herb or seasoning of choice

Heat a large skillet over medium high heat. Add coconut oil, allow it to melt and add red pepper. Cook for 2-3 minutes then add greens. Using tongs, gently toss greens while they cook. They will cook very quickly in about 2-4 minutes. Turn off heat and add avocado, seeds and season with salt and other seasonings to taste. For a vegetarian main course, add chickpeas or black beans. Serves 2-4.

I really do try not to judge when I cart spy. Who wants to be judged? It isn't fun. We all want to think we're making informed decisions and heck, if Dr. Oz said so, well then that's pretty good stuff.

But a container of fish oil isn't going to undo the damage from a diet that is deficient in nutrients and full of fats and chemicals. So back to the original question: "Can't I just take a pill?"

My answer is an emphatic, "No." Sorry. It just doesn't work that way. The supplement industry would like you to think it does. But it doesn't. Our bodies were meant to get nutrients from food. When we take supplements we look at nutrition from a reductionist point of view. Our bodies don't thrive on single nutrients. When lab animals are given nutrients without the benefit of food, they don't thrive and eventually die. **The synergistic effect of food is the key to our health.** It all works together. We don't know what the thousands of interactions are when foods break down to feed the cells, but we know which foods work best for health. A diet rich in whole, real foods, mostly plants is what we should eat for optimal health. But there are a few reasons why this is not happening.

First, we just don't eat the foods. Studies show that 50% of Americans do not eat any fruits or vegetables in a day. No fruit...no vegetables?! That's the "Big Mac®, Fries and a Coke" diet. But you say, "Wait, fries are a vegetable." Umm, in some form they used to be a potato, but in processing and frying most of the vitamin and mineral value goes away. Further, if we removed salads and potatoes from the list of vegetables, that number goes down even further. We don't eat enough nutrient dense foods.

Secondly, our foods aren't as nutrient dense as they once were. Produce is grown in soils that are barren of minerals and have been over-farmed. Chemical fertilizers are used to grow food instead of organic matter that amends the soil. The foods also travel from around the world, losing nutrients with each passing mile.

So we aren't eating the foods we need to get the thirteen essential vitamins and twenty-one minerals our bodies need. And even if we are, what if we aren't eating the right foods? Is it really so wrong to have a safeguard against a poor diet? I know even I occasionally hit a day when I'm running around, traveling, or just plain too busy to get all my nutrient-dense food. But we don't know where to go or who to ask about supplements. We don't understand what to take, so we just listen to Dr. Oz or a friend in Sam's Club. Then we pop pills without fully knowing what they do, if they'll help or if they'll harm. Why all this confusion over simple vitamins?

First, we're confused because the information comes from so many sources. Aunt Betty takes CoQ10 but an article in a magazine you read in the orthodontist's office said it wasn't proven to help anything. And your doctor said you should take a calcium supplement, but your sister told you that none of them absorb and they're made from harmful chemicals. Our sources for information are too varied. The media stirs the pot even more. When a study is done on a supplement, media sources most often report the sensational headline, yet many studies are flawed or misrepresented by the media.

On top of that, many of the studies are now being funded by the pharmaceutical industry. If you were a pharmaceutical company and an herb, vitamin or supplement could offer some relief for a condition, wouldn't you be interested in proving that it was worthless to take the supplement?

Pharmaceutical companies want to keep you from using supplements so they will fund studies to disprove their effectiveness. Supplements are not held to the same standards of regulations as pharmaceutical drugs. And this has the pharmaceutical industry in an uproar. Supplements cut into their sales. Yet, if taken incorrectly, supplements have the potential to damage health. So we turn to sources we think we can trust for information. We go to our doctors. But most medical doctors have minimal training in nutrition. Medical doctors in this country get an average of six hours of nutritional instruction. Not really what I would consider enough to be an expert. So our sources aren't reliable.

Not only are the sources of information unreliable, but so are the supplements themselves. You may even be confused by the fact that sometimes I refer to these pills as supplements and sometimes I say vitamins and sometimes herbs! They are all products to "supplement" our diets. But not all supplements are vitamins. If you take a single vitamin, I call it a vitamin. And there are 13 essential vitamins. But if you mix those single vitamins with other vitamins or herbs or cofactors or seaweed powder then I refer to those as supplements. So now that you're more confused, let's say you've decided you need a Vitamin D supplement because you've read an article in *Time Magazine* about all the wonderful powers of this nutrient. You're standing in the checkout line at your local chain drug store and bottles of Vitamin D are lined up like a brigade of soldiers ready to do battle for your longevity. So you throw a bottle in. But you get home and you read the label further. This is Vitamin D2. Didn't the article say you needed D3? Now you're confused again. And somewhere you thought you heard you should take 800IU or was it 2000IU? But this bottle is 400IU. Oh boy. The confusion about supplements continues. And the minimally informed are not the only ones affected by the lack of regulation, labeling and dosage information; I've been duped too.

As I mentioned, I supplement with Vitamin B12. I only use a few online sources for my supplements because these sites offer a lot of information and high quality products. (I will get to sources in a minute.) But I was at the mall and wandered into the shiny supplement store. Oooh, ahhh...everything was color-coordinated. Signage was clear and the salespeople were fit. This had to be an okay place to pick up my B12. The sleek interior and healthful façade kept me from doing the one thing I always do; I never read the label. When I got my bottle of B12 home, I put a dropper full of the liquid in my mouth.

Vitamin D-Rich Stuffed
Portabella Mushrooms

I go to a lot of events and have to check "vegetarian" as my entrée choice. The portabella mushroom is a popular choice for restaurants and event organizers because it sort of mimics a portion of meat. I like mushrooms because they are rich in so many different nutrients and one of those is Vitamin D. These are great to do ahead and can be popped in the oven 45 minutes before serving. Dried herbs can be substituted for fresh.

4 portabella caps

2 TBS olive oil

1 medium onion chopped

1 clove garlic minced

1 cup mushrooms chopped (use either additional portabella or any other mushroom)

1/2 zucchini chopped (about 1 cup)

1 red bell pepper chopped

1 cup chopped spinach

1/2 cup chopped fresh basil or 1 tsp. dried

2 tsp chopped fresh thyme or 1/2 tsp. dried

1/2 tsp salt

1/2 tsp pepper

1/4 cup Parmesan cheese

Vitamin D-Rich Stuffed Portabella Mushrooms

(*Continued*)

Preheat oven to 375. Wash mushroom caps and place topside down in a medium baking dish with sides. In a medium sauté pan, heat the oil over medium heat. Sauté the onions and garlic until soft and then add the mushrooms, zucchini and pepper. Cook for 5-7 minutes until soft. Add the spinach, herbs, salt and pepper. Cook until spinach wilts. Equally distribute the vegetable mixture on top of each of the mushroom caps. Top each mushroom with some of the Parmesan cheese. Cover the dish with foil and bake at 375 for 30-40 minutes or until portabellas are tender. Serves four.

Sweet...eww. And red...eww. I flipped the bottle over and was astounded! Red food dye and artificial sweetener! What!? From a fancy, sleek supplement store! I pitched the stuff and went elsewhere for my B12. But this proves a point. One supplement supplier's quality is not the same as the next. So how do you know what to buy? First you have to know what you are actually spending your money on. Let's take a look at what's in those pills!

I Want to Buy a Vitamin for $200

Vitamins and supplements can be expensive. In fact many a doctor or health care professional has used the term, "expensive urine" to describe the effects of taking supplements. If we don't need or can't use a nutrient, our bodies just get rid of it. So the point of taking a supplement should be to get a needed nutrient to your cells. Your cells recognize food as nutrients. Therefore, the best supplements you can buy are food-based and naturally sourced. These products offer the most bioavailability. This means your body recognizes them and can use them. But most supplements have low bioavailability. And definitely the supplements and vitamins sold in the super stores, grocery stores and even supplement stores are not food-based, natural sourced products. Instead, let me introduce you to the underbelly of supplements.

The most common form of vitamin supplement comes in a synthetic variety. These products are manufactured in a lab and are different than the same nutrients found in nature. Synthetic vitamins can have the same chemical constitutes, but have a different shape. This is important because some of the enzymes that break down and deliver these nutrients only work properly with a vitamin of the correct shape. This makes me think of the shape-sorting toys my kids used to play with when they were toddlers. Would the blue moon fit through the red square hole? Nope, it just wouldn't work. Yes the blue moon was meant to go in the sorting box, but it just wasn't going to get in through the wrong hole. This is one of the problems with the delivery of synthetic vitamins. When we give the body concentrated forms of synthetic nutrients, we don't always have the appropriate delivery system. Besides the ineffectiveness of delivery, the materials that make up these lab-derived products can be anything from coal tar to petroleum to acetylene gas and even sludge from industrial by-products!

Okay, stop. Picture a red pepper. **Wouldn't you rather get your Vitamins A, C, B6, K, fiber and magnesium from a crisp pepper than from sludge?**

Any chance you're taking these supplements? If you've ever taken a major vitamin brand that is advertised on TV or in magazines or if you purchase your supplements at a warehouse club or a chain store, chances are you've taken some variety of synthetic supplements. If your ultimate goal is more energy, then taking supplements that require your body's detox organs to work overtime may not be the best idea.

A second type of supplement is a natural-identical synthetic product. These nutrients are also lab manufactured but the molecular structure is identical to the nutrients occurring in nature. This process is one step up from a synthetic variety, and is more easily absorbed and used by the body. These supplements, however, almost always have other additives used either as preservatives, colors or to help them break down. These are generally never a pure product.

Naturally sourced products are higher up on the food chain of supplements. These include nutrients from vegetable, animal or mineral sources. But before they ever make it into a bottle and onto a shelf, these natural products still undergo significant processing. So even though you may be taking Vitamin D that was derived from fish liver oil, that fish liver oil still needed to go through a manufacturing process. And as you learned, the further a food is from its natural form, the less beneficial it is to your body. Many vitamins are marked natural. But in order to use this descriptive, a supplement has to be only 10% of actual natural-derived ingredients. The other 90% can be synthetic!

So is there a gold standard for supplements? Yes, and they are food-based. Makes sense, right? If you're supposed to get your nutrients from food, then shouldn't your supplements be food-based? But these manufacturers aren't usually chopping up vegetables and dehydrating them and popping them into a pill. That type of process usually results in low potency, fluctuating nutrient levels and limited shelf life. (The one exception is powders that contain dehydrated vegetables, sea vegetables, green super foods etc.) Instead, these food-based supplements are made by reacting synthetic and natural vitamins with extracts containing vegetable proteins and then making this into a supplement. And this is the closest to nature that you're going to find in a pill.

So now a couple questions may come to your mind. Where do I buy the best supplements and what should I take? I'd like to introduce you to a few supplement brands that I trust on my website at www.KathyParry.com. Click on the link that says, "Supplements I Trust." That answers the where, but the "what" to take is a bit trickier.

I'll Have What She's Having

When I was a freshman in college one of my roommates became obsessed with following me to the dining hall. "What time are you going to dinner?" she would ask and then proceed to join me as I walked down to the dining hall. But she didn't just want to dine with me; she followed me through the cafeteria line and carefully watched what I put on my tray. I noticed her tray started looking like an exact replica of mine. After about a week of this I asked her, "What's up?"

"Well, you haven't put on any weight and I have! I figured if I just ate what you ate for a while, I would lose some weight," she explained.

I didn't like being mirrored every day! It was an interesting concept, but a little stalker-ish. I told her it didn't really work that way. She was 5'10" - I am 5'0". Our body types, sleep schedules, family history, exercise habits, and social life were all different.

This mirroring gets to my point about supplements; there is not a one size fits all. There is not a one-a-day option to supplementation or nutrition. Individuals metabolize and use food differently. A 200-pound, overweight fifty-four year old man whose favorite meal is a dozen chicken wings washed down with a couple rum and Cokes may not benefit from the level of supplementation I take. He certainly has different issues going on. Recommended dosage is just that, recommended...by someone who doesn't know you. So just throwing the commercial big-brand multi-vitamin in your cart is probably not the best place to start your supplement regime.

The first step to taking supplements should be to assess what you're eating. Or maybe what you're not eating! Look at a week of a typical diet for you. Are you getting a wide variety of nutrient-dense foods? Do you eat good healthy fats that will deliver omega-3s to your cells? These foods include fish like salmon, flax seeds, avocados and nuts. Or what about Vitamin D? The vast majority of this country is deficient in Vitamin D. And milk isn't cutting it as a source because this is a Vitamin D2 source and less absorbed and used by the cells. So look at your diet. If you think there may be deficiencies, then you may consider supplementing.

Let's get back to my copycat roommate. You probably want to know what I take for supplements. I'd love to tell you, but I don't want any supplement stalkers. I really want you to think about what you may not be getting. This exercise is all part of your plan that we talked about in the last chapter. With that said, here are a few supplements that are high on my list:

Vitamin D3 – 1000-2000IU per day. If you live in a northern climate and do not continuously get 15 minutes of sun over a large portion of your body, you very well may be Vitamin D deficient.

Omega-3 – I put ground flax seed in my smoothie every morning. This is a whole food way to supplement my diet. I also take omega-3 fish oil supplements. Your cell membranes are built from fat, these membranes function optimally when they are made from omega-3 fats, rather than omega-6 fats. But the important thing with fat is the ratio. And unless you're having blood work done, you won't know your ratio of good fat to bad fat. But my advice on this is to decrease bad

The Ultimate Recipe for an Energetic Life

fats (fried foods, processed meats, snack foods with hydrogenated fats) and increase good fats (olive oil, coconut oil, avocados).

High Quality Multi-Vitamin – Okay, okay...if you really want to think that you can cover yourself with a vitamin go for it. I'm not convinced that a multi is the most optimal way to go, but I am also under the "it can't hurt" umbrella. But it must be a high quality food-based multi. See my website for suggestions: www.KathyParry.com

Trace Minerals – Most multi-vitamins don't have the trace minerals in them. These are the crazy things like copper, chromium, boron, zinc, etc. We don't need a lot of these substances, but when we are deficient metabolic functions don't work well and our energy levels drop.

What About the 312 Other Supplements on the Shelf?

If there are only four supplements I recommend, what about the rest of the shiny bottles on the shelf? This is where it all gets confusing. Shopping the supplement aisle reminds me of shoe shopping.

I like shoes. And I love DSW®. Do you know this store? Designer Shoe Warehouse. My nineteen-year-old daughter and I call it "shoe mecca." There are so many choices, so many darn...cute...choices. I try a lot on to find something that works for me. And it seems like so many will work for me. How to make a decision? I want fun shoes, I need work out shoes, I could use a new pair of black boots, and my black dress shoes seem outdated. Often I end up with shoes that I don't need. But I get sucked in by the packaging and the experience. And that is why so many of us also have a kitchen cupboard full of bottles of cute supplements. They all seem to offer something, but may not really make us feel any better.

All the other supplements on the shelf are usually designed to address specific concerns. I head to the workout shoe section at DSW because the tread on my running shoes is low. And when I head to the supplement store, I go to the liver support aisle because I like to drink wine sometimes and I want to support my liver in its detoxing. We look for specific formulas and herbals that may support our health concerns. My father has a few joint issues at age 80 so he takes glucosamine and chondroitin. And my daughter, Merritt, has cells that don't convert food to energy in her mitochondria. Her body doesn't produce the cofactor CoQ10, so I give her this supplement. The list of specific conditions that can be addressed by supplements is as wide ranging as depression to sexual dysfunction to varicose veins! If we have a problem, a supplement company is working to find a solution.

The problem with most of these remedies is the lack of scientific proof behind their claims. Don't get me wrong, I don't need a whole medical journal telling me that Triple Action Cruciferous Vegetable Extract from Life Extension® (one of my favorite supplement companies) may be good for me. Cruciferous vegetables (broccoli, cauliflower, Brussels sprouts, etc.) have some of the highest levels of cancer fighting compounds and substances that help maintain hormone balance. So an extract made from them sounds good to me. But will it really help me maintain hormone balance? I'm not sure. Should I try it on for size and see if monthly mood swings are reduced? And will my lack of cancer be a direct result of using this supplement? There's no way to know. I may just decide to eat more **Cauliflower**!

Without knowing the true benefits or outcomes of these designer supplements, we're really just self-medicating at random. And don't be fooled; supplements, especially herbal varieties, are medicinal. I had a friend who heard that St. John's Wort was good for depression. She was feeling overwhelmed and a bit down when she was outnumbered by a house full of toddlers. The long days were taking a toll on her moods.

Cauliflower Crusted Pizza

"If it isn't pizza, you can't call it that!" my kids said as I presented this to the table. Okay, so it isn't pizza in the sense that it has a wheat-based crust, but this tasty dish at least looks a bit like a favorite everyone knows. And it gives the benefit of those cruciferous vegetables!

1 head cauliflower cut into 1-2 inch pieces

1/4 cup olive oil

2 large eggs

1 tsp dried Italian herbs

1 tsp garlic powder

1-1/2 cups shredded mozzarella cheese

12 ounces pizza sauce

Favorite veggie topping

In a large pot either boil or steam cauliflower until tender, about 15 - 20 minutes. Drain the cauliflower and transfer to a large bowl. Mash the cauliflower with a potato masher or large fork until the consistency of mashed potatoes with minimal chunks. Add the olive oil, eggs and 1/2 cup of the mozzarella cheese and mix well.

She took the maximum dose...and then some. She saw some benefits from the herb as she moved through her day with an upbeat attitude. But after a couple weeks of supplementation her face started to go numb in random spots. Herbs can be very powerful. And mixing herbs and supplement blends with over the counter medicines and even

Cauliflower Crusted Pizza

(*Continued*)

Preheat the oven to 350. Lightly coat a pizza pan or rimmed baking sheet with olive oil or cooking spray. Pour the cauliflower mixture onto the pizza pan and press it flat, no more than 1/2 inch thick, mounding it up higher on the sides. Bake 20 minutes.

Remove the crust from the oven and spread on the pizza sauce, cheese and toppings. Bake until cheese melts 10-15 minutes. This is a "pizza" that should be eaten with a fork. Serves 4.

prescription drugs can set you up for unpleasant and even dangerous side effects. If you want to try supplements for specific concerns, I would again suggest that you use the highest quality supplement you can find. I recommend sources on my website with the confidence that these companies are committed to your health.

But since this is a book about energy, it may be good to look at a couple supplements that may boost energy. I stress "may." Again, a good deal of this is subjective and individual. If you only get five hours sleep each night, run around stressed out during your day and eat junk, no pill is going to give you energy at the cellular level. Cells convert usable food to energy. But here's a look at a couple supplements that may boost levels.

Energy gets used up every second of our days by our overtaxed bodies. And one area that is particularly taxed is our gut. The tract of the intestine is important in the role of energy because a majority of our immune function and nutrient absorption happen here. Got that? Nutrient absorption. And by now you should have it figured out. Our level of energy is directly related to how many nutrients we absorb. So if your gut isn't absorbing nutrients, you will lack energy. The first supplement I would recommend for increased energy is a probiotic.

Probiotics are the good bacteria that live in your intestinal tract. More microbes live in your gut than cells in your body! We need these beneficial bacteria to maintain our immune function and to absorb nutrients. They also reduce inflammation, improve digestion, eliminate waste build up and help maintain the walls of the gut. But before we go any further, I **do not** recommend getting your probiotics from a four-ounce container of sweetened, artificially flavored, sold-by-a-Hollywood-star yogurt. Probiotics in this form may do more damage than good! Look for probiotics that have at least 2 billion strains and refrigerate after opening. Probiotics do not need to be taken on a continuous basis. Generally a course of two weeks is a good rebuilding time frame. Taking a few weeks off lets your body naturally adjust levels.

Fermented foods supply probiotics naturally. These include: yogurt (plain, unflavored), kefir, sauerkraut, goat cheese, miso and a funny-tasting drink called kombucha. Kombucha is a mildly fermented beverage that has become so popular that home brewers form clubs. Try to incorporate some of these foods into your plan.

A second supplement I recommend for increased energy production is one that my daughter Merritt has taken since she was diagnosed with a mitochondrial disease. As I've mentioned, her disease is known as "the disease of no energy." The mitochondria are a part of every cell and responsible for the conversion of food into energy.

Coenzyme Q 10 or CoQ10 is required by the mitochondria to make this conversion happen. As we age our production of CoQ10 decreases. So age alone is a reason we get tired. This is why grandpa falls asleep in his chair! His cells just aren't keeping up. I recommend supplementation with CoQ10 after the age of forty.

The type of CoQ10 is important however. This goes back to a quality issue. You can walk into any random drug store or warehouse club and see a bottle of CoQ10, but the form that is usable by your cells is called ubiquinol. And you're going to pay handsomely for a bottle of high quality ubiquinol CoQ10. However, I will say that as soon as Merritt was put on this supplement, we saw her wake up and be more alert.

So there are a host of supplements out there touted to be good for energy. Be leery of many. Always, always read the label. I'm shocked at how many supplements actually contain caffeine. The best way to feel fully energetic is not from popping pills. The first few chapters of this book give you the recipe for living an energetic life. Supplements are just that, supplemental, not the real deal.

Are You Awake Yet?

When my daughter Merritt entered my life I had no idea that part of her journey would be to help others feel energetic. The wisdom I've gained caring for a child whose cells don't produce energy is worthy of sharing. When you can't get off the couch on a Saturday afternoon, I'd like you to think about your cells. Every process in the body happens at the cellular level. If your cells are not working properly, your body doesn't work properly. The best way to keep your cells working is to give them what they need and take away what they don't.

Discovering the reasons why you may lack energy will require a bit of investigation and work on your part. You're going to have to be honest with yourself. Are there changes you could make to your diet that will yield you more get-up-and-go? I'm guessing yes. What about sleep and stress? Are you making a plan to manage those? We all want to live an energetic life. Sometimes we get into such a rut of low energy, we can't imagine a way out. But even if you've been tired for years, you can begin to make changes that will affect how you feel. The beauty of regaining the energy you've lost is an engaged life: a life filled with experiences, shared with people you love, and one that leaves you fulfilled. That is the ultimate recipe to an energetic life.

Congratulations!

You made it! Thank you for embarking on this journey to a more energetic life. You get to decide the speed at which you travel. I don't doubt that if you decide to put the pedal to the metal and adopt a number of the strategies in this book, you'll feel more energetic today!

Review the chapters whenever you start getting that run down feeling. Begin implementing what you've learned and start living an engaged and vital life!

Please contact me with your success stories at Kathy@KathyParry.com. Or, post them on my www.KathyParry.com/facebook.

And I'd love to meet you! If you have a group, event, association or business that schedules speakers, please contact me to schedule your inspiring event. Learn more on page 189 and at www.KathyParry.com.

Wishing you an energetic life!
Kathy

P.S. As a **special bonus**, I've included one more chapter describing my top twenty Super Foods! For optimal energy and health, everyone should include a number of these foods in their daily diet! There are more **amazing recipes** in this chapter!

P.P.S. And are you ready for one more **FREE Bonus**? Go to www.KathyParry.com for your **FREE Chocolate Lovers Recipe Booklet**. These recipes are delicious and healthful!

BONUS CHAPTER

20 Superfoods for More Energy

Wearing a Cape Does Not Make You a Superhero

I was at my local Starbucks and a four-year-old boy came zooming through the store. His mother, pushing a baby stroller, was caught up in the serpentine line that flowed around the corner. But the little boy didn't care where his mother was, he was on a mission. As he flew by the line en route to peer through the pastry case, I couldn't help but notice his cape. It wasn't close to Halloween. But he was sporting the tell-tale sign of a superhero, a powerful red cape. I observed the boy and realized that cape had some magic. It seemed to transform him into a confident and bold little guy, willing to duck through strangers and climb refrigerated cases. But as his mother finally caught up with him, I watched him diminish. "Get down! We are not getting any treats today!" she scolded. Poor little superhero pouted off, put down by a greater power.

This scene illustrates exactly what we do to our food. We dress it up in powerful packaging, put fancy labels like natural and whole grain on it, and boldly push it past other foods. And when we do this to our food, we are given the perception that it is a superfood; a superhero of nutrition that will save us. Unfortunately, like the little boy in the cape, we find out these foods aren't very powerful. The only real foods with super powers are those in their whole, real form. They don't have to dress up to give you powerful benefits.

"Superfood" has become a trendy term. But what are superfoods? First, they don't come in packaging. They are in their real, whole forms. Superfoods are those foods that do a variety of jobs in the body. Just like superheroes, they have more than one super power. Imagine if Spiderman could only leap, but couldn't actually stick to the buildings or spin webs?

Some of the super powers that these foods have include: detoxifying, digestive aid, acid neutralizing, and anti-cancer properties, they contain high phytonutrients, and are high in specific nutrients like iron or calcium, high in essential vitamins, promote heart health, are anti-inflammatory and many more. If you want to begin a journey towards a more healthful diet that will leave you energized, you should begin to incorporate as many superfoods into your diet as possible. Challenge yourself. How many can you add in a day? In a meal?

Superfood #1: Water

Water typically isn't thought of as a food, but I haven't addressed it earlier and if you're low in it, you will not be energetic! Every function in the body is monitored and connected to the efficient flow of water in your body. And we can't begin to talk about superfoods if we can't use and digest them. Water is the starting point for the nutrients of any superfood getting to the cells. Saliva, digestive acid and digestive enzymes are all liquids made with water. Your body is 75% water. If you're not drinking water, your cells are not operating at an optimal level. The efficiency of every cell depends on being hydrated. You need the water to chew, swallow and digest. Water carries the neurotransmitters that communicate information from the brain to the cells. And of course we are cushioned by water. Our joint and muscle health are dependent on optimal levels of water.

Water is a little beyond a superfood. It is a key to life. If we are not getting an optimal level of water we can feel tired, depressed, constipated, and have muscle aches, joint pain, dry eyes and more. Our bodies give us signals when we are dehydrated, with dry mouth being one of the last! If you feel dry mouth, you need to drink water. At this point your body has already begun to draw water out of non-vital organs to give to vital functions. That means some of your organs are not operating well! To get the water your body requires, divide your weight in half, this number is the number of ounces of water you need each day. Keep a water bottle handy at all times.

Superfood #2: Garlic

Apparently garlic and I don't work well together. This is according to those who know and love me. They love me enough to tell me I smell. This is too bad. I love garlic. And garlic is a superfood. So garlic may not work for my breath, but for me, the health benefits imparted by garlic are worth being a little odiferous.

Garlic has anti-fungal, anti-bacterial, anti-viral and anti-oxidant properties. Putting odor aside, garlic has been used for centuries to heal. Besides just using garlic to fight off a cold or infection, the compounds in garlic have been studied extensively to help with heart health, cancer risk, blood pressure, reduction of cholesterol and inflammation, and combating allergies.

Unfortunately the majority of the health benefits come from raw garlic. This is not to say there are no benefits to cooked garlic, because there certainly are. But to enjoy the most healing compounds in garlic it is best to crush raw cloves and allow them to sit for 15 minutes before using them.

Superfood #3: Avocado

It doesn't happen with ice cream. Can't claim it is true with fries or butter. But this high fat food is also a superfood. Avocado is hands-down one of my favorite foods. The luscious taste that fat brings

White Bean and Garlic Dip

This is a nice change from its bean dip cousin, hummus. The white beans lend themselves to blend with almost any flavor. Lemon and tarragon seem to be very popular with my friends!

1 can cannellini beans, drained and rinsed

2 cloves raw garlic

1/4 cup fresh tarragon leaves or 1 tsp. dried

1/4 cup good quality olive oil

2 TBS Lemon juice

Salt and pepper to taste

Roughly chop the two cloves of garlic on a cutting board. Add the garlic and tarragon to the bowl of a food processor. Pulse on and off until both are chopped fairly fine. Add the beans, olive oil and lemon juice. Process until smooth. Season with salt and pepper. Serve with raw vegetables or pita wedges.

to a food is usually decadent and unhealthy. But the fat in avocados has many health benefits. The monounsaturated fats in avocados help reduce LDL cholesterol and help keep triglycerides in the blood lower. This is why it is called a good fat. Add in the hefty amount of potassium, fiber and antioxidants and yes the avocado is an official member of my superfoods list!

One cup of avocado has 23% of the recommended daily value of folate. Studies show that people who eat diets rich in folate have a much lower incidence of heart disease than those who don't. Avocados are an excellent source of glutathione, an important antioxidant that researchers say is important in preventing aging, cancer, and heart disease. Avocados have more of the carotenoid lutein than any other commonly consumed fruit. Lutein protects against macular degeneration and cataracts, two disabling age-related eye diseases.

Chop avocados onto sandwiches, eggs and salads. They also make any salad dressing thick and creamy.

Superfood #4: Flax Seed

You've probably figured out that I'm a fan of flax seed considering I start every day with this superfood in my smoothie. And why shouldn't I start my day with the power it offers? First, ground flax seeds offer omega-3 fats. These are the same fats that are in the popular fish oil supplements that people buy by the bucket at the warehouse stores. But this vegetarian option of omega-3s offers a host of additional benefits. Flax seeds also contain lignins. This substance helps to bind toxins and carry them out of your body. Flax is also high in fiber, a macronutrient that many of us are low in. Without enough fiber, digestion slows and nutrients are not efficiently absorbed.

To get the most benefit from flax seed, it must be ground. The outer hull is not broken down by normal digestion so if we don't consume it in a ground up form, we don't get the benefits of the seeds. Ground flax seed is found everywhere but it should be refrigerated after you open it so oils in it don't turn rancid.

Superfood #5: Nuts and Seeds

In my pantry is a storage container filled with a mix of power. It is a nut and seed combination I make and it is my mid-morning or three in the afternoon go-to snack. It is a mixture of pumpkin seeds, sunflower seeds, and almonds all sprinkled with some zesty spices. Although nuts are high in fat, frequent nut eaters are thinner on average than those who almost never consume nuts. Those who ate nuts at least two times per week were 31% less likely to gain weight than were those who never or seldom ate them in a study involving 8865 adults. Almonds contain riboflavin and L-carnitine, nutrients that boost brain activity and may also reduce the risk of Alzheimer's disease. Pumpkin Seeds have anti-fungal and anti-viral properties, magnesium and zinc. And sunflower seeds have Vitamin E, B vitamins and copper. Copper helps keep skin and hair healthy.

A few nuts that stand out as superfoods include almonds, walnuts and Brazil nuts. Almonds are high in monounsaturated fats, which help keep LDL (bad) cholesterol low, reducing the risk of heart disease. Almonds are also high in Vitamin E and magnesium. High levels of magnesium keep blood flow at optimal levels. Walnuts should be eaten with their papery skin intact because 90% of the phytonutrients are found in the skin. These phytonutrients have anti-inflammatory properties as well as benefits to reduce cancer risk. And finally, consider eating the big ugly Brazil nuts. You know, the ones everyone leaves in the bottom of the mixed nuts! Besides the benefits of monounsaturated fats and Vitamin E, Brazil nuts boast an ample amount of selenium. This trace mineral is important for proper function of the thyroid. It also protects the heart and liver.

Nuts and seeds should be eaten in their raw form. Sorry, no roasting or honey coating! Use nuts and seeds to top salads, in nut butter forms, ground in sauces, and even in sandwiches. Once you begin to add nuts and seeds to your favorite dishes, you'll wonder how you ever enjoyed them without the crunch!

Superfood #6: Salmon

I love to watch those video clips of grizzly bears standing in frigid streams catching jumping salmon with their mouths. Nature rarely disappoints. The ease with which these huge creatures capture their life-giving meal is phenomenal. And the bear, while scary (you know my bear stories!) is a smart animal. Wild salmon is one powerful superfood. Bears rely on these salmon to bulk up for their long winter hibernation. And we should add wild salmon to our diet, not to bulk up, but for a number of other benefits.

Wild salmon has brain and nerve benefits. Your brain is insulated with fat. The myelin sheath that keeps your brain from misfiring is made up of healthy fats like those found in salmon. So the fat found in salmon, along with Vitamins A and D, amino acids and selenium, all protect the nervous system. This omega-3 fat is also the type of fat that lowers bad cholesterol and raises good cholesterol.

But, stick to the wild salmon. First of all, wild salmon have higher levels of omega-3s because they are working harder than their farm-raised cousins. Farm-raised salmon often has artificial color added to it to give it the salmon color. In addition the condition of the water and the type of feed given to farm raised salmon is often low grade and polluted. As with all natural foods, it is best to eat salmon with the least amount of processing as possible. Avoid pre-seasoned or marinated choices as these often have artificial flavors. I was surprised to learn that one of the cheapest and easiest ways to get wild salmon is to buy canned salmon. Although not a huge fan of canned foods, canned salmon is almost always wild. It is caught in northern waters and processed very quickly at plants along the bays.

Superfood #7: Olive Oil

If you have not heard of the benefits of olive oil you may have been under a rock for the past ten years. All kinds of foods tout olive oil in the ingredient list as a selling point. Olive oil is the staple to the Mediterranean diet that gets so much attention. The fat and phytonutrient qualities in olive oil make it one of my favorite super foods. I can't prepare dinner without it.

Olive oil has been shown to lower cholesterol, cellular inflammation and blood pressure. Besides all of the health benefits, olive oil adds a delicious flavor to a variety of foods. But it is best used un-heated. Once olive oil is heated, it loses some of its beneficial properties. I still use it to cook, but it is best used for dressings, to drizzle on cooked vegetables or to add to sauces or dips.

Superfood #8: Coconut Oil

When I take the lid off my coconut oil, I always take a deep sniff. The stuff makes me want to eat a spoonful. The smell is heavenly and it produces some delicious foods! But even though it is a plant-based fat, I don't recommend fat by the spoonful. Often I have people ask, "But I thought it was a bad fat?" Nothing could be further from the truth. Coconut oil is a saturated fat, but it breaks down more easily in the body than many other fats. It is a medium chain fatty acid and unlike so many other fats, it requires less time and energy to break down. Your liver and gallbladder don't work as hard.

And when organs convert food to energy more efficiently, you stay energized longer!

Coconut oil also has anti-bacterial, anti-fungal, and anti-viral properties. It is a healing food. Studies have also shown that it increases thyroid function. And if you remember, a healthy thyroid function also leads to feeling more energetic.

Unlike olive oil, coconut oil is a perfect fat to cook with. It does add a slight coconut flavor to foods, which makes it perfect for a number of Asian-inspired foods.

Superfood #9: Tea

Okay, maybe it's been a while since you've sat down to a tea party. Unless you have a four-year-old little girl in your house, you may not have the opportunity to enjoy the ritual. But consider pouring yourself a cup of tea for your health! For centuries tea has been touted for its health benefits. But not until recently have scientific studies backed up the ancient claims.

Polyphenols in tea called catechins have been linked with anti-cancer activities. A lot of the health focus on tea has been centered on green tea because it has the highest levels of catechins. Sipping 1-4 cups of black or green tea may lower the risk of certain cancers, cardiovascular disease and Parkinson's disease. The hundreds of studies on tea point to an increased enthusiasm for its health benefits. But there is one benefit overlooked by the science, slowing down to brew, sip and enjoy a cup of tea is a great way to lower stress levels. And keeping stress hormones low is a key to feeling energetic. I encourage you to steep a cup of tea. But leave out the cookies and scones.

Superfood #10: Curcumin

A few years ago I made a sauce using the spice turmeric. The bright, golden-yellow spice splashed on my shirt and stained it. I was annoyed. But since that messy day, I've learned to respect the potent properties in vibrant turmeric powder.

Curried Lentil Salad

1-1/2 cups French green lentils

1/2 cup olive oil

3 cups water

1/4 cup wine vinegar

1 cup chopped celery

2 tsp sugar

1 cup chopped cucumber

1/2 tsp salt

1 cup raisins

1/2 tsp pepper

1/4 cup chopped purple onion

2 tsp curry powder

1/2 cup chopped cashews

Simmer the lentils in the water until tender, about 20-30 minutes. After lentils cool, add celery, cucumber, raisins, and onion. Whisk together oil, vinegar, sugar, salt, pepper, and curry. Stir together and chill before serving.

The phytonutrient (plant chemical) in turmeric that stained my shirt is called curcumin. Curcumin's big superfood properties involve its ability to interfere with cancer cell development. Cancer protection in a spice! These findings have scientists scrambling to find ways to utilize these properties to both prevent and battle cancer.

You can start protecting your cells now by simply adding turmeric to your meals. This spice is most often found in curry powders. So adding curry powder to chicken or tuna salad is an easy way to start. One of my favorite ways to incorporate curry is with lentils. This traditional Indian combination is loaded with nutrients and protein.

Superfood #11: Cinnamon

Every other day I mix a big pot of gluten-free hot cereal on the stove for my daughter Merritt. She's been eating this same cereal mixed with avocados every day for lunch for the last ten years. Kind of boring, but she loves it. And into that cereal, I always mix a couple heaping teaspoons full of cinnamon. The smell in the house is wonderful!

Cinnamon is an ancient spice that has been used for its health benefits for centuries. It is full of powerful flavonoids that plan vital roles in blood sugar regulation. It also has anti-clotting properties and anti-viral properties. A teaspoon of cinnamon mixed into some oatmeal is a great preventative measure at the first sign of a cold.

Look for some of the special cinnamons at spice stores that come from around the world. These delicious spices from China, Vietnam and Japan all have unique flavor profiles that can be equally strong and sweet at the same time. Mix cinnamon into plain yogurt, use it in marinades and dressings and even stirred into your coffee. Just don't mix it with sugar or think that certain sugar-filled breakfast cereals are healthful because they have cinnamon in them.

Superfood #12: Mango

I get it. The mango isn't that sexy to look at. It isn't cute like the raspberry or unique like the pomegranate. It's at its best when a few blemishes and brown spots cover its flesh. But don't dismiss this powerhouse. The mango is in my top 20 superfoods for a reason...or two or three. You only have to look at their deep orange color to know they are loaded with antioxidants. One small mango provides a quarter of your recommended daily allowance for Vitamin C, nearly two thirds of your daily quota for Vitamin A, and good amounts of Vitamin E and fiber. They also contain Vitamin K, phosphorus and magnesium. Mangoes are particularly rich in potassium, which can help reduce the risk of high blood pressure.

Mangoes also contain pectin, a soluble dietary fiber, which has been shown to lower blood cholesterol levels. Recently, scientists at The Institute for Food Research discovered that a fragment released from pectin binds to, and inhibits galectin 3, a protein that plays a role in all stages of cancer progression.

Superfood #13: Blueberry

The big deal about blueberries besides Vitamins C and E is the antioxidant content. Blueberries and pomegranates rank highest among fruits.

In a USDA Human Nutrition Research Center laboratory, neuroscientists discovered that feeding blueberries to laboratory rats slowed age-related loss in their mental capacity, a finding that has important implications for humans.

The compound that appears responsible for this neuron protection, anthocyanin, also gives blueberries their color and might be the key component of the blueberry's antioxidant and anti-inflammatory properties. Blueberries, along with other colorful fruits and vegetables, test high in their ability to subdue free radicals. These free radicals, which can damage cell membranes and DNA through a process known as oxidative stress, are blamed for many of the dysfunctions and diseases associated with aging.

Superfood #14: Pomegranate

When I make my lists at the holidays, one thing is always on it: Buy a pomegranate. Only available October through January, this powerhouse fruit should grace your holiday table. Multitudes of studies have been reported in clinical journals.

The pomegranate is one of the most studied fruits because of its chart-topping antioxidant properties. Higher than grapes, blueberries and even red wine, pomegranates help control free radicals. Free radicals cause damage to healthy cells as they invade, looking for a missing electrons. Most notably this "oxidative stress" effects heart health, skin and immune function.

Okay, I'll admit it. I'm vain. I first really got into pomegranate juice when I read an article that declared it "Nature's Botox®." All our organs age from oxidative stress (abundant free radicals). And our skin is our largest organ. So, when we have a high level of free radicals, our skin ages. We wrinkle. After just a few days of drinking a couple ounces of pomegranate juice, I noticed a visible difference in the lines around my eyes. If you can see this on the outside...just imagine all the good things happening on the inside!

Look for only 100% juice and don't overdo it. A few ounces are plenty. Juice of any kind quickly raises blood sugar and your insulin response.

Pomegranate Salad

Take this to the neighborhood open house, office party or family dinner. The colors are festive and the health benefits are great!

Seeds from one whole pomegranate

1/2 cup chopped dates or yellow raisins

One pear, sliced or chopped with skin on

1/2 cup chopped, toasted walnuts or pecans

1/2 cup goat cheese or feta

6-8 cups (a big salad bowl full) of mixed greens, arugula or spinach

Vinaigrette:

1/2 cup extra virgin olive oil

2 TBS red wine vinegar

2 TBS balsamic vinegar

1/2 tsp. Dijon mustard

1 TBS honey

Pinch of salt

Combine salad ingredients in a large salad bowl. Put all dressing ingredients in a glass jar with a lid and shake vigorously. Toss just before serving. Serves 8

Alternatively, for a more composed look, salad greens can be plated and pomegranate, dates and walnuts and cheese can be put on top and dressing drizzled before serving.

Superfood #15: Kale

Anyone who knows me well knows I love kale. You have probably noticed it pops up in a lot of my recipes. Kale has recently become a nationwide obsession. I walked into my local Trader Joe's on a Sunday and was looking for the kale. "Oh you're too late today," said a helpful person in produce, "Everyone on Sundays walks out with a bag of kale. We won't have more until tomorrow."

More and more studies are coming out in support of the nutrient value found in these humble leaves. Unfortunately, we stray away from greens. Too bitter, too much hassle to cook, too mushy, too green. Too bad for us because kale offers nutrients that our bodies desperately need. Our cells use the phytonutrients in green vegetables to detox, fight cancer cells, improve cellular functions and keep free radicals under control. A study at the Human Nutrition Research Center on Aging at Tufts University determined that kale offers more antioxidants than any other vegetable. It also has folate to prevent heart disease, calcium, magnesium and lutein that protects against macular degeneration.

One of my favorite ways to use kale for family meals is chopped very fine and added to sauces, tacos, and soups. My kids never know it's there!

Superfood #16: Brussels Sprouts

The oblong orbs sat sadly on my plate as I prayed for a natural disaster or at least a passing dog to take them from me. Brussels sprouts. UGH. As a child, the bowl of grayish-green cruciferous balls represented a culinary anomaly. They were cute. Cute things should taste good. But my palate had yet to decide that these nutrient-dense veggies were anything but to be avoided.

Roasted Sweet Potato and Kale Salad
with Soy Sesame Dressing

I made this salad on an October afternoon. The kale in my garden was still producing luscious leaves and I had a few sweet potatoes sitting in the cupboard. When this salad was finished, I proclaimed it one of the best salads I've ever eaten and promptly had a second bowl!

2 sweet potatoes, chopped into small cubes

1 medium onion, chopped

1 TBS coconut oil or olive oil

Salt, Pepper, and Garlic powder

1-1/2 cups edamame (fresh soy beans, also sold frozen)

4 cups chopped kale, 1/2 inch pieces

1 dried apricots, chopped

1/2 cup pepitas (pumpkin seeds)

Dressing

1/2 cup olive oil

1/4 cup red wine vinegar

1 TBS lemon juice

1/2 tsp Dijon mustard

1 TBS soy sauce

1 tsp sesame oil

1/2 tsp ground ginger

Roasted Sweet Potato and Kale Salad
with Soy Sesame Dressing
(*Continued*)

Combine all dressing ingredients in a glass jar with a lid and shake vigorously.

Preheat oven to 400. On a baking sheet with sides, place the coconut oil or olive oil. Add chopped sweet potatoes and onions. Dust the vegetables with salt, pepper and garlic powder. Roast in the oven, stirring every five minutes, for a total of 20 minutes or until tender with a bit of brown on edges of sweet potatoes. Remove from oven and let cool.

Put the edamame, chopped kale, apricots, pepitas in a medium bowl. Add the cooled sweet potato/onion mixture. Start with about 1/2 the dressing, toss the salad and add more to taste if needed.

Fast forward a few decades and I rejoice when I see the fall bounty of Brussels sprouts hit the produce shelves. Yes, my palate has redefined tasty, but also cooking methods for Brussels sprouts have gone beyond boiled and buttered. Restaurants now offer shaved Brussels sprout salads and caramelized sprouts with goat cheese. These humble cruciferous veggies have been elevated.

But besides just tasting good, the big nutrient deal with Brussels sprouts is glucosinolates. These are detox-activating compounds that are shown to fight against and even prevent cancers. Over 100 studies in the national health research database, PubMed, focus on the benefits of Brussels sprouts. And over half of these studies involve research on the cancer fighting properties of these powerhouse veggies. In another study funded by the National Cancer Institute, 20 participants were encouraged to eat 1 to 2 cups of cruciferous vegetables a day. After three weeks, the amount of oxidative stress in their body was measured. And the results? Oxidative stress in the subjects' bodies dropped 22% during the period when they were eating lots of cruciferous vegetables.

Besides these plant-based chemicals, one cup of Brussels sprouts also offers 25% of your daily fiber intake, 50% of your omega-3 and healthy doses of Vitamins C, E, A and K. Go on...if you've never picked up a package or a stalk of these cute yet mighty vegetables then this is the time!

Superfood #17: Chickpeas

Even when my pantry is bare, I always have a can of organic chickpeas. As a vegetarian, I'm always looking for easy, quick protein sources. I know that by opening a can of chick peas I can meet not only my protein requirements, but also treat myself to a long list of nutrients and phytonutrients.

I call beans the trifecta of foods. They offer three important things: protein, fiber and phytonutrients. True superfoods. And chickpeas, or garbanzo beans, are my favorite because they are one of the easiest to digest and provide more Vitamin C and nearly double the iron of other beans. Besides that, chickpeas have calcium, magnesium and potassium, all needed for bone health.

Brussels Sprouts with Fennel and Basil

A delicious main course meal, this recipe packs in several superfoods!

2 cups Brussels sprouts sliced into 3-4 slices each

1 fennel bulb sliced thin in about 1 inch pieces

1 medium onion sliced thin and cut in 1 inch pieces

2 TBS olive oil

1/4 cup water – more if needed

1 can organic garbanzo beans or cannellini beans

1/2 cup chopped fresh basil

1/2 tsp garlic powder

1/2 tsp sea salt

Dash of red pepper flakes if you like some spice

Parmesan cheese for the top

In a medium sauté pan heat the oil over medium heat. Add the Brussels sprouts, fennel and onion. Sauté ten minutes, stirring frequently. Allow them to get a bit brown on the edges. Put a lid on the pan and let cook for another ten minutes. Add water to the mixture if it begins to stick.

The vegetables need to sweat and caramelize a bit. Add the remaining ingredients, except Parmesan, and cook another five to ten minutes until flavors come together. Top with Parmesan. Serves two as a main course or 4-6 as a side.

Superfood #18: Mushrooms

When I was twelve, I discovered my love of mushrooms. We used to go to a restaurant that had amazing hamburgers. My favorite was a mushroom burger. Up until the discovery of my mushroom burger, I thought mushrooms came in creamed soup. My new culinary sweetheart launched my life-long love affair with the powerful fungi. I no longer eat the burger, but mushrooms are a staple superfood for me.

In other cultures, mushrooms have long been used for their medicinal properties. They have anti-viral and immune-boosting effects. When I feel a cold coming on mushrooms are in my arsenal of foods to eat. They are also one of the only plants that contain Vitamin D.

A mushroom found in Brazil called the Agaricus Blazei Murrill or the ABM mushroom is being studied extensively because people in this region who consume the mushroom have very little disease. The ABM mushroom was shown to cause a 3000% increase in NK or natural killer cells, a type of anti-tumor white blood cell.

Try adding a variety of mushrooms to your diet. Their earthy flavor pairs well with many foods in the fall and winter when our immune systems need a boost!

Superfood #19: Sweet Potatoes

A couple of years ago I looked at one of those national holiday calendars and realized I had been missing a major event. National Sweet Potato Awareness Month! Where had I been? Well, that led me to run a campaign called the Sweet Potato Extravaganza. It was wildly successful. Well, in my opinion. Lots of people signed up to receive two weeks of sweet potato recipes, all culminating with *The Only Sweet Potatoes I Serve at Thanksgiving.* I was interviewed on the news. Kind of a big sweet deal.

But fun aside, sweet potatoes are an awesome superfood. They contain a healthy dose of fiber, B, C and E vitamins, magnesium and the biggie, Vitamin A. One sweet potato contains the entire recommended amount of Vitamin A required for day. Vitamin A is a potent antioxidant. It protects the skin from sun damage and helps repair and restore skin. Ever notice how some very expensive eye creams tout Vitamin A as an ingredient? Vitamin A is also essential for eye health. Besides all those benefits, the sweet potato is versatile.

Superfood #20: Dark Chocolate
The Best Superfood for Last

People think the wellness lady doesn't eat sweets. You're wrong. I love chocolate. A day does not go by without chocolate melting in my mouth. I travel with chocolate in my work bag. I make special trips across town for my favorite bar. And I, a woman who shares everything with those I love, have been known to hide chocolate from my family. I can't do without it. I'm probably addicted. But, I don't have too much guilt around my chocolate habit. The bars I consume are 85% cocoa, and cocoa is the superfood.

Cocoa contains over 500 natural chemical compounds. These flavonoids are the some of the same compounds found in blueberries, green tea and red wine. These antioxidants reduce free radical damage. Dark chocolate has been shown to lower blood pressure and protect from UV sun damage. It also has anti-clotting and blood thinning properties, making it beneficial to heart health.

Of course the one thing to look out for when consuming chocolate is the amount of sugar. A regular Hershey bar has 22 grams of sugar. My dark chocolate bar has 6 grams. While I've watched a ten year old spit my chocolate into the sink, once you acquire a taste for the darker chocolate, there's no going back. Try to eat dark chocolate that is at least 72% cocoa. Stirring dark cocoa powder into yogurt and adding some stevia is a wonderful way to get the benefits of this superfood. Of course traveling with a bar of chocolate in your purse is another!

Tactics for Superfoods

I love to watch the Food Network. What foodie doesn't? In recent years I've heard the term "flavor layering" used over and over. A really good dish, according to celebrity chefs like Bobby Flay, includes complex flavors that are a result of layering a bunch of flavors from various ingredients. In various stages of making the recipe, chefs, (and home-cook-chef-wanna-bes) develop flavors by using a long list of ingredients. These are not the five ingredient meals touted by Rachel Ray.

Using superfoods to their fullest potential is a bit like developing some "flavor layering." I mean really, pretty much no one chews on a stalk of kale by itself. It's better to put it with stuff. And as you've seen from a number of my recipes, I try to layer my superfoods. Chef Flay, I call this "Nutrient Layering."

Make a list of the superfoods you like. Do a little research to find some more. My twenty foods aren't the only superfoods out there. Begin to look for recipes that incorporate more than one of the superfoods. When you make a favorite recipe, think of a superfood from the list and see if it will work well in your dish. Can your tacos take some kale? Can your muffins have some flax seed and nuts? Or could your chicken soup be enhanced with some beans? The idea of nutrient layering is easy once you decide to make the additions.

I wish you many flavorful and nutritious meals!

Recipe Index A
By Chapter

Chapter 6

Chocolate Fruit and Seed Snack Bars

Midnight Munchies Kale Dip

Five Star Crock Pot Lentil Sloppy Joes

Chapter 7

Quinoa with Roasted Tomatoes and Zucchini

Indian Spiced Chick Pea and Lentil Stew

Stuffed Acorn Squash

Spinach and Orzo Tomato Soup

Chia Seed Crackers and Red Pepper Salsa

Buffalo "Chick" Dip

Chapter 8

Blackened Wild Salmon Burger

Mixed Sauteed Greens with Avocados and Red Peppers

Spinach Stuffed Portabella Mushrooms

Cauliflower Crusted Pizza

Chapter 9

White Bean and Garlic Dip

Curried Lentil Salad

Pomegranate and Pear Salad

Roasted Sweet Potato and Kale Salad with Soy Sesame Dressing

Brussel Sprouts with Chick Peas, Fennel and Basil

Recipe Index B
By Type

Stuffed Acorn Squash

Mixed Sauteed Greens with Avocados and Red Peppers

Spinach Stuffed Portabella Mushrooms

Cauliflower Crusted Pizza

Brussels Sprouts with Chick Peas, Fennel and Basil

Fish/Chicken

Chicken Tenders with Parmesan and Herbs

Ginger Roasted Salmon with Asian Vegetables

Blackened Wild Salmon Burger

Snacks/Breakfast

Morning Wake-Up Smoothie

A Carrot is a Carrot Muffin

Mocha Almond Cooler

Colorful Berry Yogurt

Apricot Snack Bars

Chia Seed Crackers and Red Pepper Salsa

Buffalo "Chick" Dip

Desserts

Double Nutrient Dense Brownies

Chocolate Fruit and Seed Snack Bars

About Kathy Parry

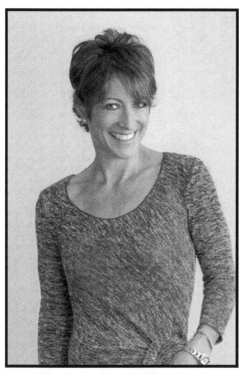

Kathy Parry – Your Real Food Coach
Author, Speaker, Mother of 4

Kathy Parry is passionate about food - real food. She helps others understand what real, whole foods are and how they affect health and vitality. Raised by parents who grew a garden full of vegetables, Kathy has long embraced a whole food diet. Food has the power to transform health and Kathy wants to share her love of eating whole, real foods with you.

With degrees in Business and Food Management, Kathy set out to change the world of food; but first she trained bankers. Feeling pressured, she gave in to the idea that "all serious people go into banking," where Kathy discovered her love for standing up in front of people as she developed and delivered training programs for a super-regional bank in the South. After leaving the world of banking, Kathy jumped at the chance to get back to her real passion and she began to sell imported and specialty foods. This immersion into food fueled her desire to encourage others to eat real food. Soon, those others she was encouraging came in the form of four children.

Pureeing organic broccoli and avoiding Happy Meals became the food activities that filled her days. But it was child number four that changed the way Kathy viewed food. After a tumultuous six months of not knowing why her child who had daily, uncontrollable seizures was not thriving, Kathy finally got answers. Merritt Joy was diagnosed with a mitochondrial disease. Her cells didn't metabolize food properly. Kathy spent the next several years becoming an expert in cellular function and received her certification in plant-based nutrition from T.Colin Campbell Program at eCornell University. Now twelve years later, Merritt Joy has never been hospitalized or suffered from any of the debilitating viruses the doctors feared. She is highly disabled, but very healthy.

While Merritt's condition could have been the flat tire that ruined Kathy's food journey, it instead became the impetus for the passion that takes her and others to places of great health and vitality.

Kathy Parry – Your Real Food Coach is Kathy's speaking and coaching business. She helps others through corporate wellness programs, event and keynote speaking and college and association programming. To learn more about how Kathy can inspire your group to live an energetic life, read the next page for details.

Choosing a Speaker is an Important Decision. Your Audience Will Thank You for Choosing Kathy Parry!

Do you have a group, association, business or event that needs to be inspired and energized? Kathy Parry shares vital information and humor from the front lines of her life to create an event that is fun, yet life-changing.

Audience members walk away with a pocket full of "ah-ha!" moments. Her energy keeps audiences engaged and her encouragement helps any willing participant start making healthful changes the second they leave the auditorium.

Kathy offers the take-away tips that audiences want and the "wow" factor and professionalism that meeting planners value.

Five Reasons Meeting, Event, and Convention Planners Love Booking Kathy Parry:

1. Experienced Speaker: Kathy has given hundreds of lectures, workshops and seminars to groups, clubs, associations and businesses.

2. Fascinating Facts: By keeping up-to-date on the most current food and health related topics, Kathy keeps audiences enthralled with information.

3. Fun and Humorous: As a mother of four, Kathy is relaxed and shares the humorous stories from her family's front lines. She is spontaneous and feeds off the audience to keep everyone engaged.

4. Real and Authentic: You'll hear the good and the bad habits that Kathy has experienced on her own journey to wellness. (Yes, she used to drink Diet Pepsi!)

5. A Powerful Coach: Kathy uses coaching techniques to inspire her audiences to make immediate changes.

To schedule Kathy for your next event:
Call 412-427-1137 or
Email Kathy@KathyParry.com

Request your speaking brochure today and sign up for a FREE Report: "Ten Ways to Stay Energized" at www.KathyParry.com.

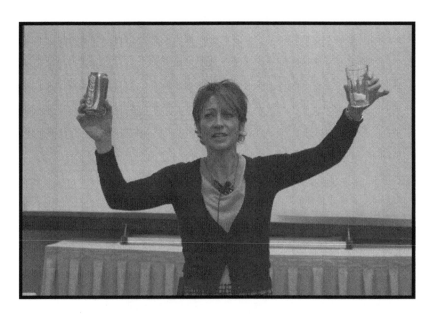

Kathy During a Keynote Presentation with Eye Opening Demonstrations!

Acknowledgements

I crave an energetic life, yet it is in the quiet moments of my life when I feel the most gratitude. So when I sit, breathe deep and think of all the gifts that have been bestowed on me, I am most grateful for the following people:

My children: Paige, JP, Graham and Merritt - Thank you for understanding your fun-loving, veggie-eating mom. I live to make you proud and I'm proud of all of you in so, so many ways! And thanks for putting up with sweet potato week.

My family: Dad, you epitomize energy and strength and you eat your veggies! Your guidance and wisdom are the greatest gifts. Heather, so many women would covet a sister like you. Tom, Marti, Bill and Caroline, David and Mo, thanks for your continued support.

My friends who never, never let me down: Bobbie, Jenny, Cindy, Susan, Mary, Linda, Maureen, Dianne, Val, Rika, Ken, Connie, Sydnee, Renee, Bryan...and so, so many more.

And the people behind the making of this book: Weston Lyon - Plug & Play Publishing, Cynthia Closkey – Big Big Design and Kathy Schenker – Schenker Graphic Design.

Made in the USA
Middletown, DE
03 February 2019